A GUIDE TO

# Specimen Management in Clinical Microbiology

THIRD EDITION

# A GUIDE TO

# Specimen Management in Clinical Microbiology

## THIRD EDITION

**J. MICHAEL MILLER**, PHD, (D)ABMM, (F)AAM
Microbiology Technical Services, LLC
Dunwoody, Georgia

AND

**SHELLEY A. MILLER**, PHD, D(ABMM)
University of California at Los Angeles
Los Angeles, California

**ASM PRESS** *Washington, DC*

Library of Congress Cataloging-in-Publication Data

Names: Miller, J. Michael (Jon Michael), 1945- author. | Miller, Shelley A., author.
Title: A guide to specimen management in clinical microbiology / J. Michael Miller, Microbiology Technical Services, LLC, Dunwoody, Georgia; Shelley A. Miller, University of California, Los Angeles, Los Angeles, California.
Description: Third edition. | Washington, DC : ASM Press, [2017] | Includes bibliographical references and index.
Identifiers: LCCN 2016053693 (print) | LCCN 2016054512 (ebook) | ISBN 9781555819613 (pbk.) | ISBN 9781555819620 (ebook)
Subjects: LCSH: Diagnostic microbiology--Handbooks, manuals, etc. | Diagnostic specimens--Handbooks, manuals, etc.
Classification: LCC QR67 .M54 2017 (print) | LCC QR67 (ebook) | DDC 616.07--dc23
LC record available at https://lccn.loc.gov/2016053693

10  9  8  7  6  5  4  3  2  1

Address editorial correspondence to
ASM Press, 1752 N St., N.W.,
Washington, DC 20036-2904, USA

Send orders to ASM Press, P.O. Box 605, Herndon, VA 20172, USA
Phone: 800-546-2416; 703-661-1593
Fax: 703-661-1501
E-mail: books@asmusa.org
Online: http://www.asmscience.org

*Section opening photo credits:* Section I (©Zaharia Bogdan Rares/Shutterstock.com), Section II (©Gotzila Freedom/Shutterstock.com), Section III (©Pongsak A/Shutterstock.com)

# Contents

**SECTION I**

## Communicating Laboratory Needs   1

## SECTION II
## Specimen Management Policies and Rationale  41

## SECTION III
## Specimen Collection and Processing  65

**Body Fluid Specimens  67**

**Gastrointestinal Specimens  77**

## Wound Specimens  141

**SECTION IV**

# Specimen Management Summary Tables  153

## References  193

## Index  199

# Preface

From syndrome-based molecular panels to total lab automation, clinical microbiology has evolved rapidly over the past 18 years since the previous edition of this book. We have witnessed increases in infections due to multidrug-resistant organisms, have overcome a major Ebola outbreak, and are currently tackling the geographic expansion of Zika virus and its potentially devastating effects. Aside from these more contemporary headliner agents, we continue to battle the threat of microorganisms that have been plaguing our world for decades, including HIV, syphilis, and influenza, just to name a few. And while the laboratory processes, diagnostic methods, and diseases may be more advanced and exotic, one unwavering aspect is the need for appropriate, well-collected specimens. In a world where we find ourselves trying to do more each day within the same 24-hour period, it is imperative that time not be wasted on correcting issues that are easily remedied with upfront attention to quality of specimens.

For some reason, clinical microbiologists seem to get more formal training in appropriate specimen selection, collection, preservation, and transport than nurses, physicians, and other medical personnel who are actually obtaining the specimens. Microbiologists can usually agree that a poor specimen, regardless of how it is transported or stored, will provide poor, even inaccurate, results for the physician. Physicians must be able to trust the microbiology laboratory to deliver accurate, clinically relevant results; so it must be emphasized that the quality of the specimen submitted for culture and, ultimately, the person selecting, collecting, labeling, preserving, and transporting it, are essential first steps to achieve this. Therefore, this book is for every member of the health care team—the partnership.

The overall aim of this edition was not to reinvent the wheel when it comes to providing guidance on specimen collection and management, because not much has changed since prior editions. Rather, it is meant to make the content more readable and accessible for its users, both specimen collectors and laboratory personnel, as well as to provide updates in specimen collection for newer methodologies (e.g., nucleic acid amplification tests) that are now in almost every laboratory. In the age of molecular testing in microbiology, the principles of specimen selection, collection, and transport are certainly no less important than they have been over the years. Close attention must be paid to the manufacturer recommendations for specimen collection and management, and unless the laboratory is prepared to validate an alternative process, one must follow these recommendations. Additionally, for labs based in the United States, the imminent threat of stricter FDA regulations on these modified tests is a reminder to us all that we must do our due diligence to prove the reliability and value in the tests we perform daily.

While the paradigm of the conventional gold standard may slowly be shifting away from cultures and organism isolation and on to more rapid, molecular-based methods, it is critical that we, as a laboratory community, continue to insist upon specimen collectors to follow collection guidelines so we can contribute what is expected of us. Anything less borders on malpractice and should be addressed before aberrant and potentially harmful results are reported. Regardless of the issue, we must remember, even in the era of decentralized labs, the specimen is not just a swab or a tube of fluid passing through our doors; it represents a sick patient, a concerned family member, and a treating physician, desperately depending on us to provide accurate, significant, and clinically relevant data. It is our mission to ensure that what comes to our lab in the form of a specimen and what leaves our lab in the form of results is of the highest quality. Please share these policies and processes with all of the medical staff involved in specimen management, share your knowledge, and spread this important information. If you don't do it, who will?

*J. Michael Miller*
*Shelley A. Miller*

# Acknowledgments

The valuable reviews and constructive criticisms of John McGowan, Robert Jerris, Mark Neumann, Ellen Jo Baron, Craig Smith, Lynne Garcia, Ben Gold, Don Finnerty, Louis Wilson, and William Reichert are greatly appreciated. We are thankful for the direct and invaluable assistance and contributions of two internationally known pediatric microbiologists, Karen Krisher and Joseph Campos. We acknowledge and appreciate the developmental work done on the summary tables by Dr. Harvey T. Holmes. We wish to thank the laboratory staff of Children's Healthcare of Atlanta, under Dr. Robert Jerris, and UCLA, under Dr. Romney Humphries, for their cooperation and willingness to participate in many of the photographs illustrating this book. We are also indebted to dozens of colleagues who have been so generous with their advice and knowledge over the years and are always working for the best outcomes for their patients—our thanks goes out to you. And finally, to the countless other microbiologists whose work in the laboratory has made significant contributions to the clinical relevance of laboratory results—we salute you.

# About the Authors

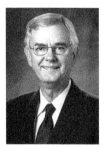 **J. Michael Miller** currently directs Microbiology Technical Services, LLC, a private laboratory consulting service. Prior to this, Dr. Miller was with the Centers for Disease Control and Prevention (CDC) for 35 years until he retired in 2011. He received his BS and MS at Northwestern State University in Louisiana and a PhD at the University of Texas Health Science Center at San Antonio. He is a Diplomate of the American Board of Medical Microbiology, a Fellow of the American Academy of Microbiology and former member of the Board of Governors, former dean of the American College of Microbiology, and holds a Clinical Laboratory Director License in Georgia and Microbiology Laboratory Director License for New York and New Jersey.

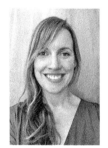 **Shelley A. Miller** completed a clinical and public health microbiology postdoctoral fellowship at UC Los Angeles and has since stayed on as a clinical instructor, assisting with clinical teaching duties and translational research projects. Dr. Miller received her BS at UC Santa Barbara and went on to complete a one-year Emerging Infectious Disease fellowship at the Arkansas Department of Health Laboratory, sponsored by the Association of Public Health Laboratories and CDC, prior to attending graduate school at UC Irvine. She is a Diplomate of the American Board of Medical Microbiology and is licensed as a technologist in both clinical and public health microbiology. Unfortunately, she has no genetic relation to the great Mike Miller.

# How To Use This Book

Since this text is intended to be used by all members of a health care team, some parts are more useful than others to particular members of the team. The book has four major sections.

## Communicating Laboratory Needs

*For physicians, nurses, specimen collectors, and laboratorians*

This section details the premises on which quality microbiology specimen management processes depend. It introduces the concepts of specimen quality and of the relationship of specimen quality to clinical relevance, but it does not detail methods for specimen management. It also outlines some of the criteria that must be adhered to by the microbiology laboratory in the interest of good laboratory practice.

## Specimen Management Policies and Rationale

*For physicians, nurses, and laboratorians*

This important section details why the microbiology laboratory must be involved in each part of the testing process, including the preanalytical, analytical, and postanalytical steps (Fig. 1). It gives the rationale for stringent standards for specimen quality and explains some of the reasons why microbiologists may reject a specimen or insist on additional information.

## Specimen Collection and Processing

*For all specimen collectors and laboratorians*

This "how to collect . . ." section is written in the Clinical and Laboratory Standards Institute format for laboratorians and is intended to help them prepare the collection portion of their procedure manuals. This section also provides instructions for any member of the medical staff involved in selecting, collecting, storing, and transporting specimens to the laboratory for analysis. Each procedure can become a part of a laboratory or nursing procedure manual on specimen collection. Included in this section are specific directions for pediatric needs.

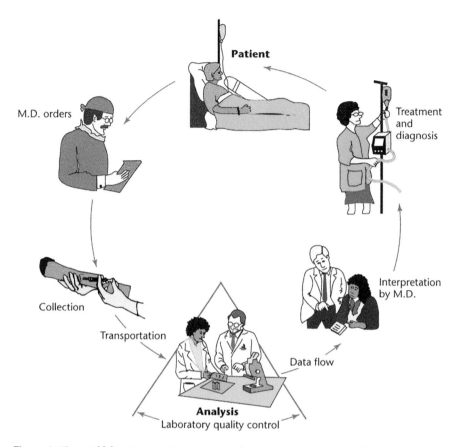

**Figure 1**  The total laboratory testing process. Laboratorians must involve themselves in all aspects of specimen management, not just the analytical process.

## Specimen Management Summary Tables

*For all personnel involved with specimen management*

This section contains summary information in tabular form for specimen management practices for bacteria, viruses, fungi, and parasites. It is to be used as a quick reference guide that can answer most questions regarding the laboratory needs for a particular specimen.

# SECTION I Communicating Laboratory Needs

*Appropriate specimen management, or lack thereof, impacts patient care in several very important ways. It is the key to accurate laboratory diagnosis, it directly affects patient care and patient outcome, it influences therapeutic decisions, it impacts hospital infection control, it impacts patient length of stay and overall hospital costs, it plays a major role in laboratory costs, it directly impacts antibiotic stewardship efforts, and it clearly influences laboratory efficiency. I would have to say this area is of critical importance to health care and to its providers and should not be taken for granted. For these reasons alone, all laboratories really need access to specialty expertise in microbiology.*

J. Michael Miller, Ph.D., (D)ABMM, (F)AAM
Microbiology Technical Services, LLC, Dunwoody, GA.

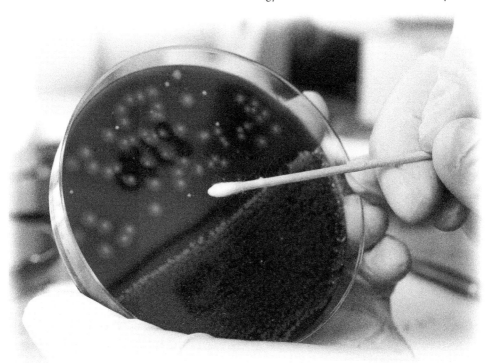

## Basic Issues

*For tissue and fluids, send the blob, not the swab.*

MELISSA B. MILLER, Ph.D., D(ABMM)
UNC School of Medicine, Chapel Hill, NC

**NOTHING** *is more important to the effectiveness of a laboratory than a specimen that has been appropriately selected, collected, and transported.*

- If specimen collection and management are not priorities, the laboratory can contribute little or nothing to patient care or related investigations. It stands to reason, then, that if laboratory data are used to supply critical information that either confirms or leads to a diagnosis and successful treatment, those involved in selecting, collecting, and transporting these microbiology specimens must understand the needs of the laboratory regarding the specimens.

- In addition, laboratorians must know the needs of the physician in order to direct their technical efforts toward providing results that are accurate, significant, and clinically relevant. Those who actually select and collect many of the specimens submitted for culture are nurses or other medical assistants, who may know the least about the needs of the physician or the laboratory. Yet it is these initial steps of selecting, collecting, and transporting the specimen that are the most critical for microbiology, whose role is to provide potentially lifesaving data.

*Open, active communication among all members of the health care team (physicians, nurses, laboratorians, etc.) is essential for optimum patient care, but communication is often difficult at best and is occasionally nonexistent.*

- Patient care is a team effort, and if one member of the team inadvertently withholds needed information from another member, the whole team suffers because incomplete information can easily lead to incomplete laboratory results. Physicians and microbiologists need to have more constructive and seamless contact and interaction with each other.

- Microbiologists act correctly and responsibly when they attempt to clarify the real needs of the clinician regarding a culture request. This may mean asking questions, suggesting equally effective but less costly alternatives, seeking additional information, or even occasionally rejecting a specimen because of improper management prior to its arrival at the laboratory.

- Often, specimens of the least clinical value require the most laboratory resources (1). The complexities of modern laboratory technology demand use of the most cost-effective methods that will provide all the information requested. For example, if one is to use a swab for collecting a specimen, choose the very best swab to use, not necessarily the least expensive.

**3**

- Microbiologists should be invited to have more input into nursing in-service training, and nurses should make an effort to understand the unique needs of the microbiology laboratory. Strategic in-service sessions that combine nursing, infection control, and microbiology staff as a team and address the needs of each health care professional can help strengthen the relationship among members of the team.

*Laboratorians must follow standards of laboratory practice just as clinicians must follow standards of patient care (Fig. 2).*

- Laboratorians work constantly to achieve and maintain standards of good laboratory practice. These standards frequently dictate the methods and limits of specimen workup and are often challenged by requests from clinicians that cannot or should not be fulfilled.
- A good laboratory, supported by its pathologist, director, or consultant, resists efforts by physicians to force it to perform an analysis that is outside the standard guidelines or will provide potentially misleading results. This resistance is a critical means of communicating; it is not a challenge to the authority of a clinician. Clearly, the physician is communicating to the laboratory a need for some crucial information about the patient.

**Figure 2** The laboratory can provide clinically significant information when skilled workers follow approved guidelines for culture workup. The laboratorian, however, must have rapid access to pertinent patient information.

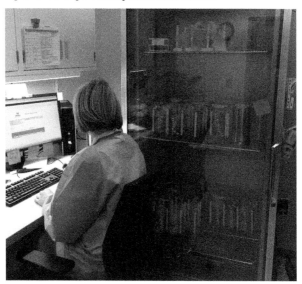

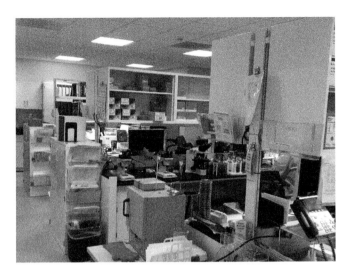

**Figure 3** Laboratory design and layout are important aspects in promoting efficient workflows that lead to improved services provided by the microbiology section.

- The laboratory must communicate what it needs in order to meet the physician's request. In fact, the laboratory's needs should be clearly documented in the section on specimen collection and handling in its microbiology procedures manual (Fig. 3).

Specimens for microbiology analysis usually contain living organisms whose recognition depends on rapid, professional specimen management. Understanding this simple concept should motivate specimen collectors to remember three important steps to accurate microbiological analysis: **SELECT, COLLECT,** and **TRANSPORT.**

1. **SELECT** the specimen from a site representative of the disease process;
2. **COLLECT** the specimen using the proper technique and supplies; and
3. **TRANSPORT** the specimen to the laboratory expeditiously or make sure that, if it is stored, storage is brief, properly done, and at a temperature that will not damage the suspected organism. Additionally, the specimen should be packaged in a container designed to promote survival of the etiologic agent and to eliminate leakage, which might pose a safety hazard and/or compromise the integrity of the results.

The health care facility's laboratory is responsible for providing detailed instructions for those engaged in specimen selection, collection, and transport. The laboratory is also responsible for in-service training of medical staff when necessary as well as responding immediately to any specimen that has been incorrectly collected or transported. Some common collection device and transport issues are outlined below in Table 1.

**Table 1** Transport concepts and solutions

| | |
|---|---|
| **Anaerobes** | Anaerobic transport tubes and vials are necessary to optimize recovery of anaerobic bacteria. |
| | Some anaerobic transport systems are available in screw-cap tubes and some in anaerobic vials; these are useful for aspirates and tissues (preferred specimens) or for swabs (not a primary choice). The containers are usually under vacuum or may have a special gas incorporated into the container to expel oxygen. |
| | For fastidious, strict anaerobes, any exposure to oxygen can be lethal and the specimen collector must be made aware of this. |
| | Anaerobic specimens often come from surgery but may come from other areas of the hospital as well. |
| **Blood cultures** | Blood culture bottles are available in a variety of sizes and volumes for adult and pediatric collections depending on the blood culture system used. |
| | Different broth formulations are available as are unique bottles for automated blood culture systems. |
| | All blood culture bottles must have their tops disinfected prior to collection using the manufacturer recommendations, and, if no recommendation is provided, the top should be subjected to the same cleansing protocol as the venipuncture site for collection. |
| *Bordetella* | Specimens for *Bordetella* testing require a minitipped swab and a nasopharyngeal specimen that would be placed into the transport medium. Molecular-based tests may require a flocked swab submitted in a special transport medium and transported at room temperature. |
| | Culture requests require special media such as Regan-Lowe to actually transport the specimen to the laboratory. These media usually need to be warmed to room temperature prior to use, so refer to the manufacturer's instructions. |
| *Chlamydia* | There are multipurpose commercially available transport media for *Chlamydia*, *Mycoplasma*, and *Ureaplasma* suitable for a variety of test methods. Follow the manufacturer's instructions with all of these transport systems. |
| | Testing by a direct fluorescent antibody assay will require specially tipped swabs for use in collecting specimens from the endocervix, urethra, conjunctiva, or nasopharynx. Some manufacturers provide collection kits containing slides for making smears at the bedside for use with immunofluorescence. |
| **Human papillomavirus** | HPV testing may require a special cervical brush, which often comes with accompanying transport medium and instructions on how to collect the specimen. |
| | Subsequent testing is usually by probe hybridization or other molecular methods and should follow manufacturer's instructions. |

| | |
|---|---|
| **Parasitology** | Fecal specimens submitted for parasitological examination require their own unique transport vials containing preservatives. |
| | A small sample of feces is placed into the transport container and sent to the laboratory for microscopic analysis. |
| | Some rapid antigen and nucleic acid-based tests are available for protozoa, and the specimen collection and transport for these tests should follow manufacturer instructions. |
| **Sexually transmitted infections** | Specimens submitted for various sexually transmitted infection testing must be carefully selected because of the nature of the etiologic agent, i.e., *Treponema pallidum*, *Neisseria gonorrhoeae*, *Chlamydia trachomatis*, *Trichomonas vaginalis*, *Herpes simplex*, and others. |
| | There are both commercially available and manual approaches to testing for sexually transmitted infections. Commercial systems will likely require a specific collection device and transport container and will provide collection instructions. If a manual method is used, the laboratory may consider a flocked swab for some collections, aspirates for others. |
| **Stool** | For bacterial pathogens and toxin analysis, specimens may be submitted in clean, nonsterile containers with lids or a screw-cap vial containing a bacterial transport medium. |
| | A sample of the diarrheal or formed stool is placed directly into the vial for transport. The diarrheal stool is the specimen of choice. |
| | Swabs may be used in pediatric patients and then placed into the tube or vial and broken off, replacing the lid and submitting to the laboratory. |
| **Swabs** | Swabs used may be cotton or Dacron wrapped or flocked. |
| | As collection devices, swabs may be incorporated into a tube containing a transport medium such as Amies or liquid Stuart's medium. |
| | Single or double swabs may be included in the transport tubes and should not have wooden shafts. Double swabs are helpful when one can be used to inoculate media and the other used for Gram stain. |
| | Other uses for swabs include tests for rapid antigens, DNA probes, yeast cultures, screening methods (e.g., methicillin-resistant *S. aureus*, MRSA; carbapenem-resistant *Enterobacteriaceae*, CRE), some viral cultures, and nucleic acid testing. |
| | Minitipped swabs are used for nasopharyngeal collection and some urethral studies. |
| **Urine** | Collection and transport of urine specimens may vary from sterile, screw-cap cups to special Vacutainer-like transport tubes, to specific devices with growth media already incorporated into the transport container. |
| | For the Vacutainer and media-containing devices, follow the manufacturer's instructions. |
| **Vaginitis/vaginosis** | Analysis for vaginitis and/or vaginosis is often assessed using automated instruments by DNA probes or other nucleic acid-based methods; these assays will require the specific collection tube or devices designed for that particular instrument. |
| | For manual analysis, vaginal swabs may be collected and sent to the laboratory for analysis by Gram stain and, in some cases, culture. |

## Selecting a Representative Specimen

*Ideally, send the specimen, not a swab of the specimen.*

KARIN MCGOWAN
Children's Hospital, Philadelphia, PA

Selecting a specimen representative of the disease process appears simple, but specimens that have been inappropriately selected arrive at laboratories daily, usually on swabs. Laboratory data generated from these specimens can be misleading and can result in an erroneous diagnosis and inappropriate therapy. Many specimens, in fact, are mislabeled or inadequately labeled. Aspirated material or material collected by needle and syringe, such as body fluids, should not be submitted on a swab. Instead, the use of a sterile tube, transport vial, or collection syringe (with needle removed) is indicated (Fig. 4). Three common examples of miscollected or mislabeled specimens are as follows.

**Wound specimens**   "Wound" is inadequate as a specimen label. Always provide the specific anatomic site. The specimen of choice is the advancing margin of the lesion, not a superficial sample from the top of the lesion or from its contents. Record whether the wound is superficial or deep (surgical). Exudate alone is usually not adequate for culture and often contains confusing commensal flora (2, 3).

**Ear specimens**   "Ear" usually indicates a specimen from a patient suffering from otitis media, in which case material on a swab is not the specimen of choice. The specimen of choice is fluid obtained by tympanocentesis, but this procedure is painful for the patient and not frequently done. Use a tiny swab only if the tympanic membrane has ruptured and is draining. Sample the draining fluid with a swab only after cleansing the external ear canal.

**Sputum specimens**   Sputum may not be the specimen of choice for diagnosing bacterial pneumonia. A blood culture, bronchoalveolar lavage (BAL), or a transtracheal aspirate (though rarely collected) is more likely to

**Figure 4**  Aspirated specimens may be transported and submitted in the syringe, as long as the needle is removed prior to sending to the lab.

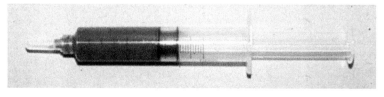

provide the etiologic agent with a higher degree of confidence. All sputum specimens are to some degree contaminated with the oropharyngeal flora. With proper instruction, patients can often provide a specimen from which true lower respiratory tract secretions can be sampled. Sputum specimens are often and correctly rejected because a microscopic examination reveals epithelial cells, which indicate contamination from the oropharyngeal flora. In such cases, the specimen should be recollected correctly.

*Commensal or normal flora provides a significant degree of "background noise" around which the microbiologist must work; some body sites have more resident flora than others.*

There are several situations in which commensal contamination may interfere with accurate interpretation of clinically relevant results and should be eliminated as much as possible before collection or avoided during collection (Table 2):

- It is specimens such as these that require great skill in culture interpretation, especially when specimen collection procedures were inadequate.

- Needle aspiration and some suction specimens tend to bypass the normal flora if the insertion site is adequately prepared. In most cases, the normal floras found in specimens need not be identified or reported if a clear etiologic agent is also present.

- Never assume that patients know what "contamination" means, and never assume that patients will do what they are expected to do regarding collection of a specimen.

**Table 2** Specimen sources likely to be contaminated

| Specimen type | Contaminating flora | Tips to avoid contamination |
|---|---|---|
| Lower respiratory tract, especially sputum | Oropharyngeal flora | Collect specimen directly in sterile container, avoiding contamination with saliva. |
| "Clean-catch" urine | Urethral or perineum flora | Carefully and completely instruct patients about how to clean themselves before urinating into the sterile specimen container. |
| Superficial wound or subcutaneous specimens | Skin or mucosal flora | Decontaminate the area, as much as possible, prior to sampling the advancing margin of the lesion. |
| "Otitis media" or "middle ear" specimens when a swab is used for collection | External ear canal flora | When possible, aspirate fluid using sterile technique. |

*The laboratory should only rarely, if ever, be given instructions to "report everything that grows" and should resist that request except in the most special circumstances.*

- Enough information is gathered at the laboratory bench from properly handled specimens to enable the laboratorian to select potential etiologic agents for further analysis and to disregard (but record) the presence of commensal or unrelated flora. If the physician presumes to be able to clearly interpret a report listing four to six isolates, the information that allows this interpretation to be made should be shared with the laboratory.
- Laboratories need a policy that confines a routine workup to a limited number of isolates while keeping the patients' and physicians' needs in mind. Usually, the more species found in a specimen, the less likely the report will provide much patient care value (1).
- For example, a laboratory may elect to work up a maximum of four species from any specimen: no more than two significant aerobes and two significant anaerobes. If the number recognized on plating media exceeds these arbitrary limits (and if no frank pathogen is present), a report such as "mixed aerobic and anaerobic flora" or "mixed skin flora" should alert the physician to the contaminated specimen and to the fact that empiric therapy may be indicated.
- Most "mixed flora" reports are due to some type of commensal contamination. The value to patient care of identifying everything that grows is questionable at best and has not been documented.
- The laboratory should of course report all frank pathogens regardless of their relation to the numbers of other organisms present.
- The laboratory should hold representative culture plates for a week after reporting so that follow-up work can be done if the physician deems it necessary.

Some criticize the decision to limit testing because such a decision is erroneously perceived to usurp the prerogative of the physician to order and interpret microbiological examinations. Most microbiologists welcome the chance to interact with physicians regarding specimen workup and reports, but, at the same time, laboratory professionals should not be pressured to provide misleading information. An American Board of Medical Microbiology (ABMM)-certified specialist is a valuable and unique resource in addressing these and other microbiology laboratory issues that involve technical and clinical correlation. The ABMM-certified microbiologist does not presume to be an attending physician but, in fact, brings special clinical and laboratory skills to bear on infectious disease diagnosis, the use of antimicrobial agents, clarity in interpretation, and support of infection control responsibilities. This specialist should be available to all microbiology laboratories to ensure technical acuity, cost-effective processes, and unique interpretive support for the staff.

## Requisitions

*It is important to put the correct patient identification on the specimen and the requisition. Valuable time is lost because of mislabeled or unlabeled specimens. As a result, the laboratory has to make telephone calls, do risk management reports, and delay plating the specimen.*

EVE BROWN, M.S., Retired

*Just as a physician needs specific and critical information from a patient's history to formulate a diagnosis, the laboratory needs specific and critical information from the physician regarding the patient and the specimen.*

- Supplying appropriate information for specimen analysis is the purpose of the laboratory requisition form, but the requisition received with the specimen seldom provides all the data the laboratory needs to interpret culture results. In fact, everything the laboratory does to analyze the specimen depends on the information included on the request form. The less information there is on the form regarding the patient and the specimen, the more difficult it is to accurately interpret culture results and relate the results to patient care.
- Computer-assisted ordering and requisition-generating systems should be designed to provide key fields that must be completed in order to submit the request transaction.

Unfortunately, the microbiology requisition may represent a weak link in the specimen management process. While electronic ordering systems are more common than paper requisitions, some laboratories may still operate with paper-based systems. In some instances, for convenience, it is the policy of some laboratories to assume that a one-page hard-copy form for all laboratory services, including chemistry and hematology, is a more efficient use of resources. On these one-page forms, microbiology services are usually allowed far too little space, and therefore too little information is provided to assist in interpreting the results for many specimens. Computer-based ordering and information systems at many institutions are able to provide a complete page dedicated to microbiology and are, optimally, designed by the microbiologist to elicit the necessary critical information.

The requisition or computer-generated submittal form, as well as the specimen container, should contain the following information:

1. Patient name
2. Patient age and sex
3. Patient's hospital/medical record number
4. Patient room number or address

5. Ordering physician information

6. Specific anatomic culture site

7. Date and time of specimen collection (critical information)

Supplemental information that, if it can be provided, would be helpful for the laboratory:

- Clinical diagnosis, special culture request, relevant patient history (e.g., travel, food, lifestyle)
- Special procedures used in obtaining the specimen
- Antimicrobial agents, if any, that the patient is receiving

**Figure 5**  Upon receipt in the laboratory, specimens are checked for proper labeling with protected health information and anatomical source information. Valuable time is lost when laboratory personnel have to follow up on specimens that are improperly labeled.

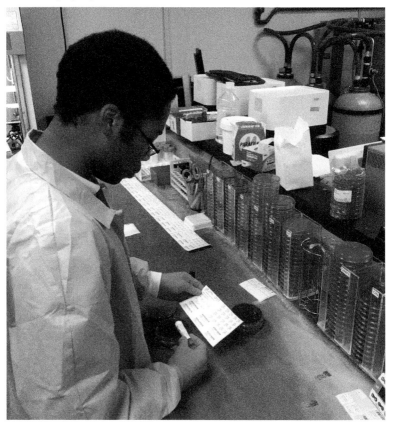

*Additional things to consider when submitting specimens:*

- All entries on the label must be legibly printed.
- The patient's first and last names should both be used to prevent a mix-up of specimens from individuals with the same surname.
- The hospital number or other designator is a valuable cross-check on the name.
- The specific culture site should be indicated, both to validate the specimen and to aid in medium selection.
- The date and hour of collection should be indicated so that culture results can be properly interpreted and efficiency of specimen management can be verified as required by licensure.
- Even though the microbiology laboratory considers each specimen potentially infectious, specimens that require emergency (stat) handling or that are known to contain a particularly dangerous pathogen (such as *Coccidioides immitis*, *Mycobacterium tuberculosis*, or a hepatitis virus) should be appropriately marked.

## Specimen Packaging and Transport

> *When you have the opportunity to send a little or a lot of material for culture, send a lot. Sending a single swab for anaerobic, aerobic, mycobacterial, and fungal culture simply proves that you believe in the atom theory, not the germ theory.*
>
> DANIEL S. SHAPIRO, M.D.
> University of Nevada, Reno, Reno, NV

*Specimens for microbiology analysis should be promptly delivered to the laboratory for accessioning and plating (Fig. 5).*

- Unlike all other sections of the laboratory, microbiology specimens contain living microorganisms. They multiply and die very rapidly. If they multiply or die during collection, transport, or storage, the specimen will no longer be representative of the disease process in the patient from whom it was taken.
- Specimens representing potential life-threatening situations, such as spinal fluid, should be quickly hand-delivered to the laboratory, when possible.
- Other specimens should be delivered in the routine manner as soon as possible after collection. Waiting until the next break, lunch hour, or shift change may contribute to a loss of viability of some pathogenic organisms, thereby potentially placing a patient's rapid recovery in jeopardy.

**Table 3** Commonly used swab types in specimen collection

| Swab type | Notes |
| --- | --- |
| Calcium alginate-tipped | Useful in the collection of specimens for detection of *Chlamydia* spp. (13). Can be toxic for viruses and some cell cultures, as well as for some strains of *Neisseria gonorrhoeae* and *Ureaplasma urealyticum*. |
| Cotton-tipped | Most nonfastidious bacteria are not affected if cotton-tipped swabs are used. May contain certain fatty acids that could interfere with the survival of some bacteria and *Chlamydia* spp. Suitable for specimens collected for *Mycoplasma* spp. taken from the vagina, cervix, or urethra. |
| Dacron-tipped | Wide range of uses including the collection of viral specimens and can facilitate the survival of *Streptococcus pyogenes*. |
| Flocked swabs | Suitable for most microbiology specimens where a swab is needed and is often equivalent to washes and aspirates. |
| Wooden-shaft | Rarely seen anymore and not recommended for routine specimen collection because the wood may contain toxic products and could inactivate herpes simplex virus and interfere with some *Ureaplasma* identification methods. |

A swab may or may not be the method of choice for collecting a particular specimen for microbiological analysis (Table 3). It is critical that specimen collectors know the appropriate device and method for collecting samples. The tips of swabs used for specimen collection are usually cotton, Dacron (a polyester), or calcium alginate. While wooden-shaft swabs are available, most swabs will have a plastic shaft (Fig. 6).

Swabs with flexible wire shafts and small tips are recommended for nasopharyngeal specimens, for male urethral specimens for diagnosis of gonorrhea, and for *Bordetella pertussis*. Plastic-shafted swabs labeled "nasopharyngeal" are not likely to contain material truly representative of nasopharyngeal flora and are most likely nasal or throat swabs.

*Factors that favor biopsy or aspiration for specimen collection (used with permission of Dr. Nancy Cornish, CDC, Atlanta, GA).*

- While swabs may seemingly be a convenient tool for specimen collection, they are suboptimal for microbiological processing as only a small amount of fluid or pus is absorbed onto the swab; release of the infected material from the swab onto agar plates is incomplete and erratic (4). In unpublished studies full-sized swabs only released about 20% of absorbed fluid onto agar plates; the performance was even poorer with mini-tip swabs, which released <10% of fluid onto the plates (Steven Dallas, Ph.D., personal communication).
- In addition, the material in swabs may be toxic to some bacteria, including important pathogens (5). Finally, should processing of the specimen be

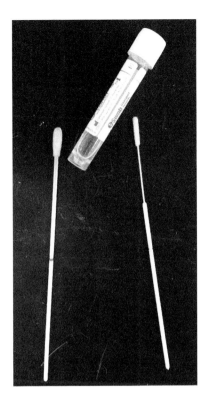

**Figure 6** Flocked swabs from commercial sources provide recommended transport containers and instructions that protect the specimen and its organisms from degradation. A variety of swabs are available for bacterial, viral, and other collections.

delayed for any reason, bacteria survive less well in swabs than in aspirated fluids or pus (6).

- With an adequate aspirate or biopsy submitted in a sterile container, the microbiology laboratory can perform all examinations the clinician may require. In addition, at some facilities all leftover tissue is frozen at –70°C for at least one month. If subsequent examination (e.g., surgical pathology) suggests a microbe that wasn't included in the original culture requests, the laboratory can retrieve tissue from the freezer for further study.

- With the miniscule amounts of material on a swab, laboratorians are limited in the number of pathogens one can culture and there is no frozen archival tissue for further study. Cellular inflammatory lesions, such as granulomas and healing wounds, are particularly difficult to sample with swabs, whereas a biopsy provides ample material for analysis.

- Direct comparisons of swabs and biopsies/aspirates from the same sources are difficult to accomplish. In most studies, even those where the authors considered the swabs acceptable, the accuracy of the swabs was only 50 to 70% compared to the reference procedure (7–9).

- When nonsterile sites, such as skin, must be traversed in order to obtain a deep specimen, the swab specimens may also be falsely positive, because colonizing bacterial flora is sampled along with the true pathogens, complicating analysis and interpretation of the results (10, 11).

*Specimen containers for transport and directions on how to use them are usually available from the laboratory (Fig. 7).*

- The potential etiologic agent suspected in the patient dictates the specific collection method and transport system that will support the viability of the agent.
- Specimens for viral culture require special transport media and holding conditions, as do specimens for *Chlamydia* and *Mycoplasma* spp.
- Fungal cultures should not be collected with a swab because of potential interference of the swab fibers with direct microscopic examination of the specimen. Swabs can be used for suspected yeast infections, however.
- Most specimen containers must be sterile because the presence of contaminating flora in nonsterile containers may lead to errors in interpreting culture results.
- Containers for feces need not be sterile but should be clean and have tight-fitting lids. If there is a question as to whether a specimen container should be sterile for a specific specimen, assume that it should be sterile.

Other useful products and devices include sterile screw-cap containers for collecting urine or sputum, which should be prepared and packaged with directions, including illustrations that can be understood by the public. Biopsy and tissue specimens can also be placed in these sterile cups, although "biopsy" samples sometimes tend to be smaller than "tissue" samples. To keep these tissues moist, a small amount of nonbacteriostatic saline can be added to the cup rather than wrapping the tiny pieces of tissue in gauze. Sterile petri dishes can be used to transport hair or skin scrapings to the mycology laboratory. Commercial transport devices for *Neisseria gonorrhoeae* such as the Jembec system, which employs $CO_2$ tablets, may provide better results than $CO_2$-containing bottles, especially for courier transport. Bottles may not have consistent amounts of $CO_2$, and improper manipulation during inoculation can cause a loss of the atmosphere.

*Specimen testing should be strategic and not a shotgun approach.*

- Some physicians are worried about overlooking an improbable diagnosis, and so they ask that multiple tests be run on the same specimen. If enough specimen is present, several tests can be performed, but the patient care value of "shotgun" culture requests must be questioned.

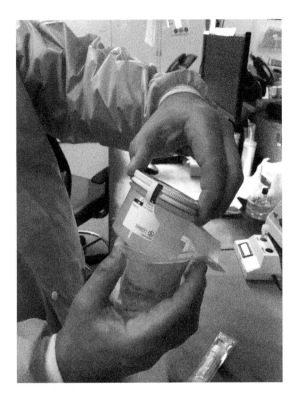

**Figure 7** Sterile cups with screw-cap lids can be used to transport a variety of specimens.

- More information from culture results (multiple isolates) is not necessarily better information. If too much laboratory information is produced, misleading information will have been forwarded to a physician who may already be perplexed about the clinical diagnosis. Consultation between the laboratory and the clinician is in order.
- There are new genetic-based multiplex test systems that can quickly provide helpful analysis of specimens by searching for multiple pathogens at once. These have a valuable place in laboratory diagnosis but require rational application and workflow design.

The microbiology section focuses on infectious disease diagnosis and is different from other sections of the laboratory. Ours is a science of interpretive judgment which is impacted at both the preanalytical and analytical steps in the specimen analysis process and, as such, requires stricter adherence to specimen management principles than, perhaps, other sections of the general laboratory. Maintenance and manipulation of living organisms require processes very different from those used in chemistry and hematology. Attention to the details of specimen selection, collection, and transport unique to these organisms is required of all members of the health care team involved in contact with the specimen. Laboratory safety must be a first priority of laboratory administration and employees, with the goal of protecting ourselves and our colleagues from a laboratory-acquired infection. Never shortcut laboratory safety (12).

## Virus, Rickettsia, Chlamydia, and Mycoplasma Transport

*Because of the advances in technology over the past few years, viral and chlamydial disease diagnosis has become a prospective science rather than a retrospective one.*

- In many facilities, viral culture is being discontinued and replaced by rapid, accurate genetic approaches to diagnosis or with other rapid assays, all of which have been critical components in positive patient outcomes.
- For viral diseases, the method of specimen collection usually dictates successful analysis whether by culture, nucleic acid testing, or other means.

*Methods and media used for bacterial transport are inappropriate for virus and chlamydia transport (13).*

- Viral transport media (VTM) are designed to prevent drying, maintain viral viability during transport, and prevent the overgrowth of contaminating bacteria. Many formulations contain either Eagle's minimum essential medium or Hanks' balanced salt solution along with fetal bovine serum or bovine serum albumin (BSA). VTM can be prepared in-house or purchased commercially. There is little evidence in the literature that one type of VTM is better than another.
- Liquid-based transport systems contain a protein (BSA, gelatin, or fetal bovine serum) and a combination of antimicrobial agents in a buffered solution. Viruses are NOT inhibited by antibacterial drugs. Tissue for viral analysis can also be placed in this type of medium. A buffered sucrose-containing transport system (2SP) can be used for virus and for chlamydiae transport; the antimicrobics present in the 2SP are not inhibitory to chlamydiae.
- A transporter system containing human newborn foreskin fibroblasts is commercially available and is useful for recovery and early detection of cytomegalovirus and herpes simplex virus. Because of the cells, however, this system has a limited shelf life and is useful only for viruses that grow in fibroblasts.
- *Rickettsia* diagnosis is usually accomplished by serology at public health or reference laboratories or by polymerase chain reaction (PCR). Isolation of *Rickettsia* requires a blood sample. A sucrose-phosphate-glutamate transport medium containing BSA can be used for rickettsia, mycoplasma, and chlamydia transport (14).

*Key points (13, 14, 34)*

Most specimens for viral analysis should be taken within 1 to 3 days of symptom onset when virus concentration is at its peak; waiting 7 days or more may result in nonproductive results, particularly for culture.

In virtually all cases where a specimen is submitted for viral analysis, it should be selected and collected in a manner that reflects the target organ that often manifests the classic symptoms of the viral disease.

If specimens for viral analysis arrive at the laboratory in a Stuart's or Amies bacterial transport system, the swabs can be transferred to a liquid VTM system.

If a swab must be used to collect a specimen, remember that viruses require cotton or Dacron swabs but not alginate swabs. Alginate impairs recovery of enveloped viruses (e.g., influenza virus, herpesvirus), can interfere with fluorescence-based assays, and can inhibit PCR. Additionally, swabs with wooden shafts or those containing charcoal should not be used when collecting specimens for viral diagnosis.

Manufacturers of probes, amplification systems, and enzyme immunoassay antigen detection systems often recommend or supply specific transport media and/or swabs for the collection and transport of specimens that have demonstrated reliable performance when tested in their systems. If the manufacturer has received FDA approval for their test when the particular media and/or swab is used, it is important to submit specimens using the approved specimen collection device; if a different device or medium is used by the laboratory, it must be validated by the laboratory prior to use.

## Transportation Policy

1. All specimens must be ***promptly*** transported to the laboratory, preferably within 2 h of collection, unless being sent to an off-site laboratory (Fig. 8).

   *If processing is delayed, specimens for bacterial agents can be stored under the conditions specified in the specimen collection tables in section IV. These storage conditions also serve as suggested conditions for transport by courier.*

2. In general, do not store specimens for bacterial culture for more than 24 h (Table 4). Viruses, however, usually remain stable for 2 to 3 days at 4°C (13, 14).

   *Specimens for viral analysis should not be frozen unless transport will be delayed, at which point freezing at –60°C or –70°C or on dry ice is recommended, never at –20°C.*

**Table 4** Storage conditions for various transport systems and suspected agents[a]

| Preservative[b] | Held at 4°C | Held at 25°C |
| --- | --- | --- |
| No preservative | Autopsy tissue, bronchial wash catheter, intravenous CSF, lung biopsy material, pericardial fluid, sputum, urine (all) | CSF (bacterial agents), synovial fluid |
| Anaerobic transport | | Abdominal fluid, amniotic fluid, anaerobic cultures, aspirates, bile, cul-de-sac, deep lesion material, IUD for *Actinomyces* spp., lung aspirate, placenta (cesarean section), sinus aspirate, tissue (surgery), transtracheal aspirate, urine (suprapubic aspirate) |
| Direct inoculation of media | | Corneal scraping, blood cultures, *Bordetella* spp. (RL, BG), *N. gonorrhoeae* (Jembec system), vitreous humor |
| Aerobic transport media | Burn wound biopsy material, *Campylobacter* spp., ear (external), *Shigella* spp., *Vibrio* spp., *Yersinia* spp. | Bone marrow, *Bordetella* spp., cervix, conjunctiva, *Corynebacterium* spp., ear (internal), genital cultures, nasopharynx, *Neisseria* spp., *Salmonella* spp., upper respiratory cultures |

[a]CSF, cerebrospinal fluid; IUD, intrauterine device; BG, Bordet-Gengou medium; RL, Regan-Lowe medium.

[b]Stuart's, charcoal-impregnated swabs originally formulated for *N. gonorrhoeae* transport; Amies, modified Stuart's but with charcoal incorporated in medium instead of swab; Cary and Blair, similar to Stuart's but modified for fecal specimens and with pH increased from 7.4 to 8.4.

3. Optimal transport of clinical specimens, including anaerobic cultures, depends primarily on the volume of material obtained.

   *Submit small amounts within 15 to 30 min of collection; biopsy tissue can be maintained for up to 20 to 24 h if stored at 25°C in an anaerobic transport system (15).*

4. Environmentally sensitive organisms include *Shigella* spp. (which should be processed immediately), *N. gonorrhoeae*, *Neisseria meningitidis*, and *Haemophilus influenzae* (which are sensitive to cold temperatures).

   **Never refrigerate** *spinal fluid, genital, eye, or internal ear specimens (aspirates) (16) or specimens suspected of containing these agents.*

5. Transportation of clinical specimens and incubating cultures from one health care facility or laboratory to another, regardless of the distance, requires strict attention to specimen packaging and labeling instructions (13, 17, 18).

*Materials for transport must be labeled properly, packaged, and protected during transport, and courier vehicles must also be marked and designated as carrying biological agents.*

Department of Transportation regulations are available on the Internet (http://www.dot.gov). Generally, courier transport conditions should follow those listed under "Storage" in the tables in section IV.

### Shipping specimens or cultures

When a culture of an etiologic agent is to be prepared for shipment, a dual-cylinder system is required (Fig. 9).

1. The culture or specimen should be placed in a screw-capped tube or leak-proof container that is clearly labeled.

**Figure 8** The physician may need some clinically relevant information within 30 min to 1 h of specimen arrival. Final reports may require 24 to 72 h for completion.

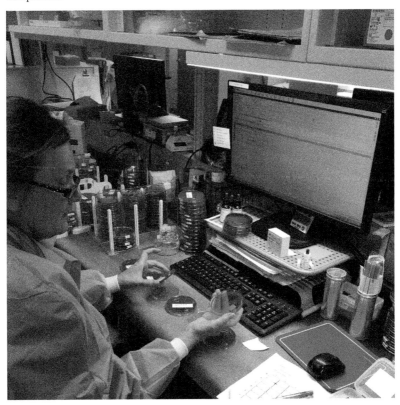

2. The lid is then sealed with waterproof tape. This tube is wrapped in absorbent packing material and inserted in a secondary shipping tube that has soft packing in the bottom to protect the specimen tube from breakage.

3. The requisition form or paperwork accompanying the specimen is wrapped around the outside of this secondary container or is written on the outside of the secondary container.

4. The secondary container is then placed in a sturdy shipping container and labeled for mailing and marked with a biosafety notice.

5. Both the shipper and consignee's name, address, and telephone number must be on the outer and should be on the inner containers.

Further information on shipping can be obtained from the Office of Health and Safety of the Centers for Disease Control and Prevention (http://www.cdc .gov/biosafety/), from the regulations on Interstate Shipment of Etiologic Agents (42 CFR, Part 72), and the Department of Transportation Hazardous Materials Regulations (49 CFR, Parts 171 to 180).

**Figure 9**  Packaging and shipping. Image courtesy of Centers for Disease Control and Prevention. http://www.cdc.gov/vhf/ebola/pdf/ebola-lab-guidance.pdf.

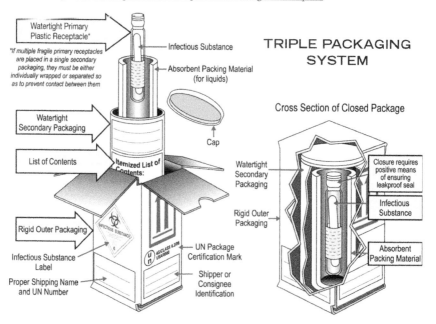

## Color-Coded Vacuum Tubes

Vacutainer-like tubes are occasionally submitted to the laboratory for microbiology processing. Little recent information on the survival rates of microorganisms transported in some of these color-coded tubes is available, but it is important to know and inform clinicians and nurses that special microbiology tubes are obtainable. Table 5 describes these color-coded tubes and their intended use.

If a specimen arrives in an inappropriate container, contact the physician immediately, explain the discrepancy, and ask for another specimen. Provide information regarding appropriate collection and transport. If the specimen from an inappropriate container must be analyzed, an addendum to the report should be added stating something like the following:

*"Specimen was submitted in an inappropriate transport container which may interfere with recovery/detection of organisms; results should be interpreted with caution."*

## Catheters Often Used in Medical Procedures

Microbiology laboratories frequently receive catheters or catheter tips for culture to determine the presence or absence of a potential etiologic agent associated with the catheter. Interpretation of culture results may be misleading, however, because of the difficulty of distinguishing etiologic agents from the commensal flora obtained from the removal site.

- For venous or arterial catheters, an accompanying blood culture is always helpful and recommended.

**Table 5** Color codes for vacuum tubes

| Color | Anticoagulant in tube | Intended use |
| --- | --- | --- |
| Black | Sodium citrate | Determination of sedimentation rate |
| Light blue | Citrate | Coagulation studies |
| Brown | Sodium heparin | Lead determination |
| Gold | Clot activator | Serum separator |
| Green | Lithium heparin | Chemistry, cytology |
| Light green | Lithium heparin | Separation of plasma |
| Gray | Oxalate-sodium fluoride | Glucose studies |
| Lavender | EDTA | Hematology |
| Red | None | Obtaining serum |
| Yellow | Sodium polyanethol sulfonate | Microbiology studies |

- Urinary catheter (Foley catheter) tips are not cultured because it is virtually impossible to remove the catheter without contaminating the tip with the urethral flora, complicating interpretation of growth.
- In almost all cases, bacteria associated with the catheter are encased in a biofilm, and they may be protected from elution onto a culture plate because of their close association with the biofilm.

Any catheter type may become colonized or contaminated and be a source of seeding the contiguous site with organisms. *Removal of the catheter may be the only way to facilitate the elimination of the source of infection.*

- For indwelling urinary catheters, urine must be taken only from the sampling port of the catheter after meticulous preparation of the port. **Urine should never be cultured from the collection bag.** Urine obtained by a straight catheter from women is usually a good sample for culture if attention to site preparation has been accomplished and aseptic collection is successful.
- Venous and arterial catheters are removed from the patient, and the distal tip of 1 to 4 in. is aseptically cut and placed into a sterile cup or tube if semi-quantitative culture is to be performed or placed into a tube of sterile saline or broth and hand-carried to the laboratory. Unmoistened catheter tips dry quickly and may injure organisms.

A partial list of catheters and their uses is shown below.

**Angiographic**   Used to inject contrast dye to visualize the vascular system of an organ. May be named according to the site of entry and destination, e.g., femoral-renal and brachial-coronary.

**Arterial**   Inserted into an artery as part of a method to monitor blood pressure of critically ill patients. May also be used for X-ray studies of the arterial system or to deliver chemotherapeutic agents into the arterial supply of tumors.

**Balloon tip**   A catheter with a balloon at the tip to inflate or deflate while the catheter is in place to create, enlarge, or block a passageway.

**Bozeman-Fritsch**   Slightly curved double-channel catheter with several openings at the tip.

**Broviac**   A right atrial catheter similar to a Hickman catheter but with a smaller lumen.

**Brush**   A ureteral catheter with a fine brush tip that is passed endoscopically into the ureter or renal pelvis and used to brush cells from the surface of suspected tumors.

**Cardiac**   A long, fine catheter used to pass through a peripheral blood vessel into the chambers of the heart under fluoroscopic control.

**Central venous**   A long, fine catheter inserted into a vein to administer parenteral fluids, antibiotics, or other therapeutic agents into a large blood vessel. Is also used to measure central venous pressure.

**Condom**   An external urinary collection device that fits over the penis. Used to manage male incontinence.

**DeLee**   Used to aspirate meconium and amniotic debris from the mouth and nose of newborns.

**Double-current**   A double-lumen catheter.

**Double-lumen**   A catheter with two channels, one for injection and one for aspiration. Also may be called a two-way catheter.

**Elbowed**   A catheter bent at an angle near the tip and mostly used in association with cases of enlarged prostate.

**Eustachian**   Used to inflate the eustachian tube.

**Female**   A short, straight catheter for passage into the female bladder.

**Fogarty**   A balloon tip catheter used to remove arterial emboli and thrombi from major veins and to remove stones from biliary ducts.

**Foley**   An indwelling catheter held in place in the bladder by a balloon inflated with air or liquid at the tip. Usually has three lumens: one for inflating the balloon, one for irrigation and sampling, and one for draining the urine.

**Groshong**   Single or double lumen (with an external port) inserted into the right atrium. Unlike the Hickman or Broviac catheter, this catheter has a distal valve to prevent blood backflow, thus eliminating the need for clamps.

**Hemodialysis**   Used in the subclavian, internal jugular, or femoral vein for arteriovenous access for hemodialysis.

**Hickman**   A right atrial catheter for long-term administration of antimicrobials, total parenteral nutrition, or chemotherapeutic agents through the venous access. May be a single- or double-lumen catheter.

**Indwelling**   Designed to be held in place in the urethra, e.g., the Foley catheter.

**Malecot**   A tube with an expanded tip used for gastrostomy feedings.

**Nasal**   A soft, flexible rubber or plastic catheter with holes in the distal tip; used to administer oxygen.

**Oropharyngeal**   Same as a nasal catheter.

**Pezzer's**   A self-retaining catheter with a bulbous extremity.

**Prostatic**   A catheter with a short, angled tip.

**Robinson's** A straight urethral catheter with two to six holes to facilitate drainage when blood clots may clog one or more holes.

**Subclavian** Inserted into the subclavian vein and manipulated into the right atrium, serving as a central venous access.

**Swan-Ganz** A soft, flow-directed catheter with a balloon tip for measuring pulmonary arterial pressure. Also called a French Swan-Ganz catheter.

**Tenckhoff's** A silicone catheter permanently inserted into the abdominal cavity in dialysis patients for infusing dialyzing solution during peritoneal dialysis.

**Texas** A trademark for a commercially made condom catheter.

**Toposcopic** A miniature catheter that can negotiate tiny vessels to deliver chemotherapy directly to brain tumors.

**Tracheal** A catheter with small holes in the tip used to remove fluids and exudates during tracheal suction.

**Ureteral** A long tiny-gauge catheter designed to be inserted directly into a ureter.

**Urethral** Any catheter inserted via the urethra into the urinary bladder.

**Winged** A soft catheter with little flaps on each side of the tip to hold it in the bladder.

## Specimen Priority

Specimens should always be processed as soon as possible after they arrive at the laboratory. To expedite the process of specimen management, the laboratory should have a method of prioritizing the handling of specimens. Generally, specimens can be classified into one of three groups: *urgent, routine, and elective.*

### Urgent

Urgent specimens represent potentially life-threatening illnesses requiring immediate attention (usually without regard to the location of the patient within the hospital) so that some preliminary information can be forwarded to the submitting physician within 30 min to 1 h of specimen arrival or first result of culture. Some facilities, as a local decision, may elect to have all specimens from bone marrow transplant patients and those on immunosuppressive therapy be considered urgent. Specimens with urgent priority (stat specimens) are:

| | |
|---|---|
| Blood | Regardless of location |
| Spinal fluid | Regardless of location |
| Transtracheal aspirate | Regardless of location |
| Eye specimens (endophthalmitis) | Regardless of location |

| Pericardial fluid | Regardless of location |
| Amniotic fluid | Regardless of location |
| Lower respiratory tract specimens | From intensive care units (ICUs) |
| Surgical specimens | From ICUs |
| Joint fluids | If septic arthritis is diagnosed |

## Routine

Routine specimens are submitted from patients at no immediate risk of life-threatening sequelae, but they represent a potentially important infectious event requiring diagnostic confirmation or preventive observation. Specimens with routine priority include:

| Throat specimens | Regardless of diagnosis or location |
| Pleural fluids | Regardless of diagnosis or location |
| Burn specimens | Regardless of diagnosis or location |
| Eye specimens | Regardless of diagnosis or location |
| Urine, catheter | If sepsis is diagnosed |
| Urine, any | From ICUs |
| Genital specimens, female | Obstetrics/gynecology or surgery if sepsis or septic abortion is diagnosed |
| Surgical specimens | From operating room |
| Lower respiratory tract specimens | If pneumonia is diagnosed |
| Peritoneal fluid | If peritonitis is diagnosed |

## Elective

Elective specimens are those whose processing is handled as expertly and judiciously as that of other specimens but whose results may be more confirmatory than part of an emergency diagnostic procedure. All specimens other than those listed above as urgent or routine specimens are elective. Table 6 offers suggestions on prioritizing specimens for workup.

## Priority Issues

*After an initial diagnosis, testing the same specimen type from a given patient on a daily basis usually provides little useful clinical information but it may be a local decision to do so.* In general, if symptoms persist beyond initial culture, a 3-day interval for submitting repeat specimens appears optimal for detecting pathogens that may have developed resistance or that are currently involved in the infection (19). *Staphylococcus aureus* and *Pseudomonas aeruginosa* may require more frequent reexamination. Another exception is specimen analysis for *M. tuberculosis*.

**Table 6** Specimen priority for processing[a,b]

| Specimen | Replica limit | Priority |
|---|---|---|
| Blood | 3/24 h maximum | Urgent |
| Body fluids (not spinal fluid) | | |
|    Amniotic fluid | None | Urgent |
|    Pericardial fluid | None | Urgent |
|    Joint fluid (arthritis) | None | Urgent |
|    Bone marrow | None | Routine |
|    Peritoneal fluid | None | Routine |
|    Pleural fluid | None | Routine |
|    Ascitic fluid | None | Elective |
|    Bile | None | Elective |
|    Transudate | None | Elective |
|    Joint fluid (not arthritis) | None | Elective |
| CSF | None | Urgent |
| Environmental specimens | | |
|    Intravenous fluid | | Routine |
|    All others | | Elective |
| Eye | None | Routine |
| Genital, female (not anaerobe) | | |
|    Endocervix | 1/day/type | |
|    Vaginal | 1/day/type | Ob/Gyn ....................................Routine |
|    Urethra | 1/day/type | |
|    Placenta | 1/day/type | Sepsis or abortion ................................Routine |
|    Vulva | 1/day/type | |
|    Lochia | 1/day/type | All other ....................................Elective |
|    Perineum | 1/day/type | |
| Genital, female (anaerobe) | | |
|    Placenta, cesarean section | 1/day/type | |
|    Endometrium | 1/day/type | ICU .......................................... Urgent |
|    Uterus | 1/day/type | |
|    Culdocentesis | 1/day/type | Sepsis or abortion ................................Routine |
|    Fallopian tube | 1/day/type | |
|    Cervical aspirate | 1/day/type | Ob/Gyn/OR..........................................Routine |
|    Ovary | 1/day/type | |
|    Bartholin's gland | 1/day/type | All other locations ...............................Elective |
| Genital, male | 1/day/type | Elective |
| Postmortem specimens | | Elective |
| Lower respiratory tract | | |
|    Tracheal | 1/day | ICU .......................................... Urgent |
|    Bronchial | 1/day | Pneumonia ..........................................Routine |
|    Sputum | 1/day | All other locations and diagnoses ......Elective |
|    Transtracheal aspirate | None | Urgent |
|    Lung biopsy | None | Urgent |

| | | |
|---|---|---|
| Upper respiratory tract | | |
| Throat | 1/day/type | Routine |
| Nose | 1/day/type | Elective |
| Oral | 1/day/type | Elective |
| Ear | 1/day/type | Elective |
| Sinus | 1/day/type | Elective |
| Nasopharynx | 1/day/type | Elective |
| Stool or rectal | 1/day | Elective |
| Surface specimens | | |
| Burn | 1/day/type | Routine |
| Cyst | 1/day/type | Elective |
| Decubitus | 1/day/type | Elective |
| Exudate | 1/day/type | Elective |
| Laceration | 1/day/type | Elective |
| Lesion | 1/day/type | Elective |
| Paronychia | 1/day/type | Elective |
| Skin | 1/day/type | Elective |
| Stoma | 1/day/type | Elective |
| Suture | 1/day/type | Elective |
| Ulcer | 1/day/type | Elective |
| Vesicle | 1/day/type | Elective |
| Surgical specimens | | |
| Abscess | 1/day | |
| Aspirate | 1/day | |
| Biopsy | None | |
| Bone | None | |
| Clot or hematoma | 1/day | |
| Drain | 1/day | |
| Exudate | 1/day | |
| Fistula | 1/day | ICU .......................................................... Urgent |
| Intravenous catheter | 1/day | |
| Prosthesis | None | OR..........................................................Routine |
| Pus (purulent exudate) | 1/day | |
| Stone | None | Other locations .....................................Elective |
| Tissue | None | |
| Wound | 1/day | |
| Urine | 1/day | ICU .......................................................... Urgent |
| | | Other locations .....................................Routine |

[a]CSF, cerebrospinal fluid; Ob/Gyn, obstetrics and gynecology; ICU, intensive care unit; OR, operating room.
[b]Adapted from Ellner (40) with permission of the publisher.

*A policy for handling and reporting stat or urgent specimens is not only essential for good patient care but is also required by the Clinical Laboratory Improvement Amendments (CLIA) of 1988.*

- The policy should specify which specimens are considered urgent by the microbiology laboratory, whether or not they are labeled as such.
- Optimum use of stat testing is of critical importance to patient care, but indiscriminate use of the stat request can lead to expensive and unnecessary laboratory testing.
- Carefully selected quality indicators used by the laboratory to evaluate efficiency can constantly monitor appropriate use of the stat request. Likewise, physicians must understand that the laboratory is obligated to locate and call them 24 h/day to report requested stat results.

If a specimen is considered urgent, the results must be rapidly and accurately obtained and communicated to the requesting physician. These tests should require that the results be telephoned to the physician, and information on contacting the physician should be on the requisition or in the hospital or laboratory information systems (HIS or LIS).

- Find the physician or a designee, even if he or she must be called at home. Leaving a message with a nurse or with anyone other than the requesting physician or designee may interfere with the immediate care of the patient.
- Record in a telephone log book, on computer specimen records, or in the LIS that the results were telephoned and include the date of the call, the physician spoken to, the message given, and who made the call from the laboratory.
- Telephone messages about results from specimens other than urgent requests can, at the discretion of laboratory policy, be given to another medical staff member as long as the information regarding the call is recorded as described above.

## Specimen Rejection Criteria

*Just because you can culture something doesn't mean you should!*
Eileen M. Burd, Ph.D., D(ABMM)
Emory University Hospital, Atlanta, GA

The procedure manual for every microbiology laboratory is required by licensure agencies to include a section on the rejection of specimens submitted for examination. These rejection criteria are designed to prevent the production of inaccurate data and to ensure the safety of laboratory personnel.

*Remember:* Rejection of a specimen is not a repudiation of the health care provider who submitted it, nor is it an indication of the absence of infection. It is simply a request for a new specimen that will provide the clinically relevant information necessary for good patient care. In fact, unless the rejected specimen container is leaking and exposing laboratory personnel to potential danger, it should be held in the laboratory until the physician is notified and another specimen is requested.

At times, specimens arriving at the laboratory have been improperly selected, collected, or transported. If these specimens are processed, they may provide misleading information that can lead to a misdiagnosis and inappropriate therapy. *In the laboratory, when controls reveal a test to be potentially inaccurate, the results of that test cannot be reported. Remember that a specimen can be out of control.*

- Because providing clinically relevant results requires quality specimens, the laboratory must adhere to a strict policy of specimen acceptance and rejection. **The microbiology laboratory should flatly reject specimens of poor quality.** Table 7 lists some of the criteria used for specimen rejection.
- If the physician, for any reason, insists that the results for an improperly selected, collected, or transported specimen be reported, the laboratory must include in the report a statement explaining the potentially compromised nature of the results. Clearly, the clinician should know all the relevant data the laboratorian knows about each specimen.

**Table 7** Criteria for rejection of a specimen

| Problem | Action |
|---|---|
| Improper or no label | Telephone the physician or nurse. Have someone come to the laboratory and identify the specimen before it is processed. If no answer, call or page the physician. Repeat the call during each subsequent shift and again after 24 h. Process the specimen but do not publish the results until the physician has been consulted. |
| Prolonged transport<br>Urine: >1 h at room temperature (unpreserved)<br>Stools for trophozoites: >1 h since collection<br>Gonorrhea specimens: >1 h without transport medium | Alert the submitter to the discrepancy and request a repeat specimen. Note the problem on the report: "Received after prolonged delay." |

*(Table continues on next page)*

**Table 7** Criteria for rejection of a specimen *(continued)*

| Problem | Action |
| --- | --- |
| Improper container (nonsterile) | Do not process. Call the submitter and request a repeat specimen. If the physician insists on processing, alert the supervisor and indicate the discrepancy on the report. |
| Leaking container | Do not process sputum, blood, or viral specimens. Call the submitter for a repeat specimen and autoclave the leaking container. For other specimens, call the submitter and ask for a repeat specimen. Otherwise, note the discrepancy on the report. Protect the laboratory staff. |
| Oropharyngeally contaminated | Do not report (or process). Indicate the discrepancy on the report. Request another specimen. |
| Obvious foreign contamination | Alert the submitter to the contamination discrepancy on the report. Request another specimen. |
| Duplicate specimens submitted at same time | Select the one best-quality specimen for culture. Report by adding a note to the report form. |
| Duplicated specimens submitted on same day for same request (except blood) | Place the specimen in a refrigerator. Call the submitter and indicate the duplication. Culture on request only and note the request on the duplicate specimen result. |
| Specimen unsuitable for culture request, e.g., anaerobe request with aerobic transport | Call the submitter and indicate the discrepancy. Request a proper specimen for the work requested. |
| Quantity not sufficient | For blood: if <5 ml from an adult, inform the submitter and request another specimen. Process but note the problem on the report. For other specimens: if quantity is not sufficient for multiple requests, call the physician and determine the priority of requests. |

For various reasons, all of which will result in the production of questionable data, some frequently submitted specimens are generally unsuited for microbiological examination, and they are listed in Table 8. Transport and holding temperatures are often critical to the survival of etiologic agents (20). Each member of the health care team should be aware of these nonproductive or misleading types of specimens and should resist submitting them for microbiological analysis. In addition, the laboratory may receive requests for anaerobic bacteriology studies that are inappropriate because the specimen may provide misleading results. Table 9 lists both appropriate and inappropriate specimens for anaerobic studies.

**Table 8** Specimens to be discouraged because of questionable microbial information

| Specimen type | Action |
| --- | --- |
| Superficial oral and periodontal lesion, swab[a] | Request tissue or aspirate |
| Decubitus, swab | Request tissue or aspirate |
| Varicose ulcer, swab | Request tissue or aspirate |
| Burn wound, swab | Request tissue or aspirate |
| Superficial gangrenous lesion, swab | Request tissue or aspirate |
| Perirectal abscess, swab | Request tissue or aspirate |
| Bowel content | Do not process |
| Vomitus | Do not process |
| Foley catheter tip | Do not process |
| Colostomy discharge | Do not process |
| Lochia | Do not process |
| Gastric aspirate of newborn | Do not process |

[a]Specimens from oral lesions are best processed by laboratories equipped to provide specialized microbiological techniques for detecting and enumerating specific pathogens.

**Table 9** Suitability of various clinical materials for anaerobic culture

| Acceptable material | Unacceptable material |
| --- | --- |
| Aspirate (by needle and syringe) | Bronchoalveolar washing, not protected |
| Bartholin's gland | Cervical swab |
| Bile | Endotracheal aspirate |
| Blood | Endocervical swab, contaminated |
| Bone marrow | Lochia |
| Bronchoscopic, protected brush | Nasopharyngeal swab |
| Culdocentesis specimen | Perineum |
| Fallopian tube | Prostatic or seminal fluid |
| IUD[a] for *Actinomyces* spp. | Sputum, expectorated |
| Ovary | Sputum, induced |
| Placenta, via cesarean section | Stool[b] or rectal sample |
| Sinus aspirate | Throat swab |
| Stool, for *C. difficile* | Tracheostomy aspirate |
| Surgery, swab | Urethral |
| Surgery, tissue | Urine, bladder or catheter |

*(Table continues on next page)*

**Table 9** Suitability of various clinical materials for anaerobic culture *(continued)*

| Acceptable material | Unacceptable material |
| --- | --- |
| Transtracheal aspirate | Urine, voided |
| Uterus, endometrial aspirate | Vagina or vulva |
| Urine, suprapubic aspirate | Wound, superficial/surface |

*[a]*IUD, intrauterine device.

*[b]*There are a few exceptions, namely, botulism (especially infant botulism), *Clostridium perfringens* foodborne disease, and *C. difficile* antibiotic-associated pseudomembranous colitis; some malabsorption syndromes may require detection of overcolonization of the upper intestine.

*Submitting multiple specimens from the same patient for bacteriological analysis within the same 24-h period is not recommended.*

- Generally, no more data are gathered from two or three daily throat or wound specimens from the same patient than from the first, properly collected one.

- Duplicate orders often prove to be clerical errors that are costly to the patient and take up unnecessary laboratory time. However, to rule out infection with some organisms, two or three consecutive negative specimens (submitted one per day) must be demonstrated. Conversely, some pathogens, such as *Giardia lamblia*, may be present in feces in such low numbers that, if only one specimen is examined microscopically, the agent might be missed. Therefore, three specimens, one every other day, should be submitted to confirm this diagnosis if microscopic examination is used. One specimen, however, may be adequate for enzyme immunoassay or molecular tests.

## Rejection Statements or Addenda to Laboratory Reports

*Remember, you are treating patients, not laboratory requisitions; if a result does not make sense to you, consult the laboratory director.*

BRUCE HANNA, Ph.D., D(ABMM)
Bellevue Medical Center, New York, NY

It is appropriate, necessary, and required that laboratorians add a statement to any report to explain the potentially compromised nature of the results if a specimen was improperly selected, collected, or transported, or had to be rejected for any other reason. Often, the bench microbiologist can determine from culture results, Gram stain results, and accompanying patient information that some type of explanation or statement regarding the status of the specimen or the interpretation of the results is in order. The purpose of the statement is only to alert the clinician to any potential problem or interpretive information that might have a clinical impact on the patient. The suggestions presented here are statements that the laboratorian might select to accompany the laboratory report. All statements used and the circumstances of their use should be approved by the laboratory director and listed in the procedure manual.

## Selected Statements To Be Used When Inappropriate Conditions Occur

**When certain isolates are not worked up.** "Organisms from this body site are not routinely processed because their identification either provides no relevant clinical information or offers misleading results."

**A problem involving preanalytical handling is evident.** "These results may or may not be clinically significant because the specimen was improperly selected, collected, or transported to our facility."

**Miscellaneous circumstances.** "These results may or may not be accurate because

- the organisms identified are of questionable clinical significance."
- the specimen was improperly collected."
- the specimen was improperly transported."
- there is heavy contamination with normal flora that interferes with the growth of potential pathogens."
- the specimen was/was not refrigerated prior to shipment."

**Additional information for the physician.** "The literature has shown a correlation between the isolation of *Clostridium septicum* from blood and a possible underlying leukemia, lymphoma, or carcinoma of the large bowel," or "The literature has shown a correlation between the isolation of *Streptococcus bovis* from blood and a possible malignancy of the gastrointestinal tract."

**Damaged transport container.** "This test was canceled because the package was received damaged and the contents may have been contaminated."

**Epithelial cells seen on Gram stain of a wound.** "Results of a Gram stain evaluation of this specimen suggest that superficial contamination is abundant and that culture will therefore provide misleading results. Large numbers of squamous epithelial cells were present, indicating surface contamination of the specimen."

**Gram stain indicates evidence of superficial contamination.** "Specimen is unacceptable for anaerobic culture. Routine aerobic culture pending. Please consult the microbiology laboratory if clinical considerations warrant further processing."

**Gram stain results suggest commensal flora.** "Gram staining of the clinical specimen suggests that the organisms reported are probably commensal flora."

**Selective susceptibility test policies.** "Susceptibility testing is not routinely performed on this organism because of its predictive response to empiric therapy. The drugs of choice may include _____."

**Susceptibility test done on an organism for which no disk or minimum inhibitory concentration (MIC) interpretive standards exist.** "This susceptibility report provides only quantitative MIC results. There are no criteria by which to interpret these results as susceptible (S) or resistant (R). Depending on the antibiotic, successful therapy may result if the selected antibiotic can reach MIC level in the affected tissue for a period of time or levels of eight times the MIC in the infected body site of an immunocompetent host. Consult pharmacy or infectious diseases."

**Reporting culture results for sputum shown by Gram stain to be unacceptable.** "Because of the large numbers of oropharyngeal squamous epithelial cells seen in the Gram stain of this sputum sample, the results may not be clinically relevant. Interpret with caution."

**Physician demands results for otherwise inappropriate specimen.** "These results are reported by special request of the attending physician and may or may not reflect an accurate etiology."

## Specialty Testing

All clinical laboratories have limits of expertise. Reference laboratories and specialty laboratories (specializing in difficult or esoteric diagnostic tests) should be used when this limit of expertise is reached or when the sophistication of the test ordered is beyond the capability of the laboratory. Molecular diagnostics, using PCR, rRNA sequencing, next-generation sequencing and other advanced procedures, may not be currently available as routine tests in some laboratories, but they offer accurate results for many common and uncommon organisms.

*To accommodate the special needs of difficult cases, a specialty or reference test menu should be made available to all laboratory clients.*

- This menu should list the tests offered, the laboratories that perform them, estimates of turnaround time, and cost confirmations.
- This same menu should be included in the laboratory procedures manual, where it should also provide directions for packing and shipping specimens to the reference site, if shipping is not coordinated by the laboratory. Ideally, this resource should be updated every 6 months because new products and tests continue to appear.
- A written log or electronic record should be maintained for all "send-out tests." The log should contain the patient's name or identifier, the physician's

name, the test requested, the site doing the work, the date the material was submitted, the date the results were received, and the time the results were sent to the physician. *Keep in mind that the report must indicate that the test was performed by a referral laboratory and must be identified on the report form by name or by a code available to the authorized requester.*

- CLIA regulations specify that the local laboratory must maintain either the original report from the referral laboratory or an exact copy for its records.

## Environmental Samples

Environmental sampling and culture is a specialized field and is as complex as collecting and processing clinical specimens from patients. Therefore, many clinical microbiologists are unfamiliar, unprepared, and not appropriately certified for the unique sampling methods and culturing requirements for environmental samples. Clinical microbiology technologists may need training in this area, and the laboratory should establish a quality control program specific to environmental analysis. In addition, state certification of laboratories is often required for certain water and wastewater testing.

*Collection of environmental specimens in health care institutions is not routinely recommended because, in the absence of direct epidemiologic data linking an environmental source to an active outbreak, culture results may be misleading. Additionally, environmental testing is often regulated by agencies other than CLIA, so a clinical laboratory should therefore acquire proper certification prior to performing such tests. CDC guidelines can be found in MMWR 52:1–42.*

- Although agents of outbreaks may be deposited and found on environmental surfaces, there is little evidence suggesting that these surfaces actually transmit the organism to patients, nor may the organisms be present in sufficient numbers to cause disease, especially in immunocompromised populations.

- The primary means of transmission of agents of disease is by the hands of health care personnel, patients, and visitors. Appropriate hand washing remains the best way to prevent most institutionally acquired infections.

Caveats to environmental sampling:

1. *In the United States, the three most common nosocomial infections are surgical site infections, urinary tract infections, and pneumonia. None of these infections is easily acquired or transmitted by touching inanimate objects or by breathing contaminated air. Therefore, routine sampling of air, water, or fomite surfaces often provides little information on how to prevent the transmission of infections.*

Reusable medical instruments and ventilators may be inadequately cleaned and disinfected, allowing an organism access to a compromised patient.

In addition, water used in some patient care procedures may not have been adequately disinfected, thereby exposing patients to organisms capable of surviving in water after inadequate disinfection or within biofilms attached to the lumen of tubes or catheters used in medical procedures.

2. *The clinical microbiologist must recognize that organisms isolated from the environment may not exhibit optimal or typical growth on enriched media such as blood and chocolate agar commonly found in the laboratory and may not be identified accurately by some commercial identification systems.*

Organisms that are viable in water have adapted to an environment depleted of nutrients and may require special incubation conditions and a chemically defined medium such as R2A on which to grow.

Water can be filtered through a 0.45-μm-pore membrane filter, and the filter can be enriched in broth or placed directly on the surface of the agar. Standard plate counts can also be done.

Currently, the only recommendation for routine culture involves water used in renal replacement therapy (hemodialysis, hemofiltration, and hemodiafiltration). In this case, the medium recommended for culture is trypticase soy agar without blood, standard methods agar, standard plate count agar, or the equivalent. Water for hemodialysis should contain no more than 200 CFU of bacteria per ml.

If the laboratory is asked to test potable water, most states require that testing comply with their own or with federal standards. In these instances, the laboratory will probably have to be certified by the state to process these samples.

3. *Organisms collected from surfaces frequently cleaned with soap or disinfectant may be viable but inhibited by the residual disinfectant picked up by common collection procedures.*

A neutralizing agent in transport solutions or in media may be required to facilitate the growth of such organisms.

4. *Air sampling for detecting indoor fungi such as* Aspergillus *spp. or bacteria such as* Legionella *spp. is difficult and complex, as is the interpretation of data collected.*

There are no guidelines for indoor air analysis that can be used to show a causal relationship to disease outbreaks.

In areas of the United States where humidity is high, one is more likely to experience the presence of *Aspergillus* spp. or other fungi in the air, in air-handling systems, and even as a frequent and annoying source of medium contamination in the laboratory.

Where an air-handling system is involved, frequent surface disinfection with fungicides or bleach only temporarily relieves the symptoms. The root problem often remains in the air-handling system, which may require professional servicing.

Concentrations of spores can change unpredictably by orders of magnitude within a few hours during a day. A powered air sampler for quantitative measurement of air volumes is a useful method for sampling air. A laboratory may only be able to document a baseline level of air contamination and then periodically monitor the critical patient care areas where transplant and severely immunocompromised patients are housed.

## Hand Wash Specimens

Results of sampling the hands as a source of nosocomial agents may direct infection control personnel to the source of spread of an outbreak. Sterile swabs are commonly used to collect hand surface specimens but may provide an inadequate sample. A special miniature gauze sponge, a commercial Handi Wipe, or rinsing hands in 200 to 300 ml of broth contained in a plastic bag may provide a more definitive means of looking at the microbial flora of the hand. A sample procedure is listed below. Hand sampling should be done only during an outbreak and only if infection control personnel have implicated the hands as a possible source of transmission. Only those personnel linked by epidemiologic data should be tested.

**If the laboratory is inexperienced in environmental sampling and culture, it is recommended that the use of a consultant be considered or that an outside specialty laboratory provide specimen collection information and technical assistance.**

If the samples are processed in-house, tests can be done on an elective basis and need not be performed during the busiest time of the day.

*Example of a hand-sampling procedure:*

1. A sterile wipe premoistened with 0.02% Tween 80 is used to scrub the palmar and digital surfaces, and the wipe can be placed in a sterile cup or bag for transport to the laboratory.

2. In the laboratory, 120 ml of sterile 0.02% Tween 80 solution is added to each cup containing a wipe, and the cup is placed on a shaker for 15 to 30 min.
3. After agitation, 0.1-, 1.0-, and 50-ml aliquots of fluid are filtered and cultured by the membrane filtration technique.

## Laboratory Reports

Detailed instructions on how to complete and submit microbiology laboratory results are not given here. However, a few issues deserve mention.

- Laboratory reports must be sent promptly only to the authorized person who will use the test results or to the laboratory requesting special studies.
- Copies or duplicates of all preliminary and final reports must be held for 2 years. Immunohematology reports and pathology reports must be held for at least 5 and 10 years, respectively.
- CLIA does not require that instrument printouts be posted on the patient's chart, but these printouts must be maintained as part of the record retention requirements of the laboratory.

The laboratory doing the test must be identified on the report. Even when hospitals consolidate and there is one central laboratory for most microbiology testing, with some testing done by associated hospitals, the specific testing laboratory must still be identified on the report to the physician. The laboratory reporting policy should address the following issues:

- Legibility of the report
- Confidentiality of the report, including the security of the laboratory information system, who has access to the report, and how unauthorized users are kept out
- An expert consulting mechanism to assist in the interpretation of results. An ABMM-certified microbiology consultant is recommended and is a wise investment for laboratories without the services of a doctoral-level clinical microbiology specialist.
- Provision, where appropriate, of reference ranges or critical results that may indicate the need for special attention or life-threatening values
- Explanation, on the report, of the potentially compromised nature of the results

*Clinicians: Know what you are going to do with results. You are responsible for review and action.*

Robert Jerris, Ph.D., (D)ABMM
Childrens Healthcare of Atlanta, Atlanta, GA

# SECTION II Specimen Management Policies and Rationale

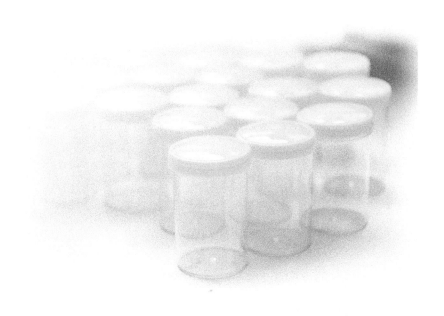

In cooperation with selected members of the medical staff or laboratory clients, the laboratory should formulate a policy for specimen management that supports both good medicine and good laboratory practice. This policy should be documented, and a copy of it should be distributed to all users and clients of microbiology laboratory services. Part of the policy should be a carefully prepared, fact-supported manual on how to collect and handle specimens. It is important for nurses and clinicians to understand the needs of the laboratory regarding specimen collection and handling. In addition, the policy should address the special needs of the laboratory and the rationale for these needs. Laboratory leaders should be prepared to provide in-service training on specimen collection and management policies to medical and nursing staff and others who collect specimens for microbiology. This section discusses simple policy statements and includes the rationale for each policy in italics.

## Collection Times

*Include the time of specimen collection on the requisition. Without it, one may not be able to interpret results.*

Patricia Charache, Ph.D., (D)ABMM
(Deceased)

1. The optimal times for specimen collection must be based on both the type of infectious disease process and the ability of the laboratory to process samples. Laboratories are usually better staffed and therefore better able to receive and process specimens during the daytime hours.

   *The microbiology laboratory may not be well staffed during evening and late-night hours.*

   *Samples collected late in the evening often do not produce adequate growth by the next morning. However, provisions must be made to handle and report urgent specimens during "off" hours, and consultation with supervisory personnel is highly recommended.*

2. Twenty-four-hour specimen collections for culture should be discouraged, and such collections should be accepted only after consultation with the microbiologist or pathologist.

   *Pathogens that appear at their highest concentration in first morning secretions will be diluted by added material.*

   *Stored samples are very likely to be overgrown with contaminants. Improved laboratory culture techniques preclude the need for large volumes of samples.*

3. First early-morning sputum and urine samples are optimal for recovery of acid-fast bacteria, fungi, and other pathogens in adults. Samples collected at other times are acceptable.

   *Early-morning secretions are more concentrated and therefore more likely to contain large numbers of the etiologic agent.*

   *Children under 7 years of age cannot reliably collect early-morning specimens. The majority of specimens from this age group are randomly collected, and therefore there are circumstances where collection on three consecutive days may be required to optimize retrieval of organisms, especially from gastric aspirates.*

   *First morning urine specimens from children who are not toilet trained are probably no better than randomly collected specimens.*

4. The timing of blood cultures should be determined by the clinical condition of the patient. Physicians should always indicate the collection schedule. A maximum of three cultures per 24 h is usually sufficient to diagnose most cases of septicemia. Newer culture systems and culturing of larger blood volumes may reduce the number of cultures needed. In many cases, two draws from two separate sites obtained at the same time may be adequate.

   *In endocarditis, typhoid fever, brucellosis, and other uncontrolled infections, bacteremia is continuous, and thus the timing of collection is less critical. In other infections, bacteremia is intermittent and may precede the onset of fever by an hour, making collection timing important.*

   *In acute febrile episodes, two draws of at least 10 ml of blood each from separate venipuncture sites allow immediate initiation of therapy. The recovery rate after three negative cultures per 24 h is extremely low except in cases in which a sudden fever spike is observed; then, drawing of an additional blood sample may be indicated.*

   *In pediatric populations, the collection of more than one blood culture in a 24-h period is determined by the size of the child and access to a suitable collection site. A volume of ≥0.5 ml is acceptable, although 1 to 5 ml from children younger than 5 years old is desirable. Refer to the manufacturer's recommendations for adequate collection volumes.*

   *Small volumes of blood from children should never be rejected. Notify the physician that a delay in detection may be anticipated because of the small volume cultured.*

5. Unless the laboratory routinely processes such specimens in-house, the following procedures should be done only after consultation with the pathologist or microbiology supervisor, and if the specimens are to be tested, the protocol should be published in the procedures manual.

**a.** Viral cultures, unless the tests are done routinely. Many viral specimens are now routinely tested by nucleic acid amplification and culture is seldom done in community hospitals.

**b.** Tests of serum-killing power or antibiotic assays of blood

**c.** Dark-field examination for spirochetes or other bacteria

**d.** Special blood cultures for recovery of fungi

**e.** Recovery of *Chlamydia, Rickettsia, Leptospira,* or other unusual organisms

**f.** In pediatric patients, testing for *Bordetella pertussis,* respiratory syncytial virus antigen detection, rotavirus antigen detection, and blood culture for *Malassezia furfur.*

*These requests often require the use of special laboratory equipment and the selection of enriched or selective media not routinely stocked in the laboratory. Nucleic acid tests are now used routinely by many facilities or are available at reference laboratories.*

*Samples often must be collected at specific times or in special ways to ensure optimal recovery of microorganisms or to produce results that can be interpreted in relation to therapeutic regimens.*

*Physicians bear the responsibility for informing the laboratory that an unusual infectious disease is suspected. Laboratory personnel should be consulted to determine whether any special techniques or collecting devices will be needed.*

## Collection Procedures

*Obtaining a good specimen is the clinician's responsibility. Generating good test results is the laboratory's responsibility. When these are combined, a negative test can be as helpful as a positive one.*

EILEEN M. BURD, Ph.D., D(ABMM)
Emory University Hospital, Atlanta, GA

**1.** All specimens must be collected in appropriate sterile containers. If samples will be delayed in processing or are being sent to reference laboratories, a transport medium must be used.

*If the container is not sterile, results may be erroneous. It is the responsibility of the laboratory to see that sterile containers of suitable leakproof construction are made available to physicians or ward personnel.*

*Specimens for viral testing should be available and the manufacturer's instructions must be followed for using the collection apparatus and the viral transport medium.*

2. Samples for anaerobic cultures are best collected by aspirating abscess fluid with a sterile syringe and needle and then injecting the aspirated fluid into an anaerobic transport vial. Although not a method of choice, syringes (with the needle removed and discarded) can be capped with the needle cover and submitted for culture. The submission of swabs for anaerobic culture is discouraged, but if they must be used, they should be immediately placed in suitable anaerobic transport packets and pushed into the agar plug.

   *It is important to carefully protect species of anaerobic bacteria from the killing effects of atmospheric oxygen and desiccation.*

   *The chances for recovery of an anaerobe are enhanced when the specimen is protected from any contact with atmospheric oxygen, as much as possible, before inoculation in the laboratory.*

   *The incidence of serious anaerobic infections is limited in pediatric populations. In this group it may be important to consider the collection of stool and blood for the diagnosis of infant botulism and food-borne intoxication caused by* Clostridium perfringens.

3. Blood, not sputum, may be the specimen of choice for diagnosing bacterial pneumonia. Sputum samples for culture must contain lower respiratory tract secretions as evaluated by Gram stain. The mouth should be rinsed with water or the patient should be asked to gargle; dentures should be removed immediately before the sample is collected. Patients must be instructed to take two to three deep breaths and then cough deeply.

   *All sputum samples are contaminated to various degrees with oropharyngeal secretions. Expect some sputum specimens to be rejected because of normal oropharyngeal flora detected on the screening Gram stain.*

   *Mechanical rinsing of the mouth immediately before expectoration reduces the number of commensal bacteria.*

   *Induced specimens or transtracheal aspirations are recommended for adult patients who cannot produce sputum. A bronchoalveolar lavage may be more productive than sputum.*

   *In pediatric populations, only older children and adolescents can be expected to provide adequate sputum specimens for analysis. In infants and younger children, secretions aspirated from the trachea or bronchi are more often submitted for the diagnosis of bacterial pneumonia.*

   *Nasopharyngeal swabs can be submitted for the diagnosis of pertussis and neonatal chlamydial pneumonia.*

   *Nasopharyngeal aspirates should be submitted for the diagnosis of respiratory viruses that cause laryngotracheobronchitis (croup), acute bronchitis, bronchiolitis, and pneumonia.*

4. Bronchoalveolar lavage (BAL) specimens are better than bronchial washings for the diagnosis of pneumonia. Both should be processed as soon as possible after they are collected. BAL may be the specimen of choice when an uncontaminated sputum specimen cannot be easily collected. Currently, there is no documentation supporting the use of an enrichment medium for delayed transport of such specimens for the isolation of *M. tuberculosis*.

*Some microorganisms that may infect the respiratory tract, such as* Haemophilus influenzae, *are susceptible to drying or low temperatures.*

M. tuberculosis *specimens should be sent unenriched to a reference laboratory. Cetylpyridinium chloride-sodium chloride is an in-transit decontaminating solution that has successfully preserved* M. tuberculosis *in sputum specimens for days while killing most contaminating organisms. If PCR is to be performed, a portion of the sample without decontaminating solution should be sent as well.*

*BAL specimens are difficult to collect from pediatric patients because of the small lumen of the bronchial tree in children and infants.*

5. The collection of clean-catch urine samples must not be left to chance. Ideally, the specimen should be collected with the assistance of a nurse or aide and always after the patient has been given specific instructions. Do not assume that a patient knows how to do what is expected. Use pictures to explain the collection procedure.

*Since most laboratories perform routine colony counts on urine samples, meticulous care must be taken in specimen collection if valid results representative of bladder urine are to be obtained. In females, there is a great potential for contamination of the periurethral area by vaginal or bowel flora.*

*If patients are to collect specimens unattended, specific verbal and written instructions will help ensure the collection of a good specimen. It may be appropriate to read the instructions to the patient, particularly if there is a language barrier. It is recommended that these instructions be printed on a card for the patient to use during the collection procedure. Instructions should be available in the predominant languages of the area. Illustrative drawings are helpful.*

*The requisition should indicate whether the patient is symptomatic or asymptomatic. This information allows the laboratory to more correctly interpret the numbers of organisms present in the specimen and provide clinically relevant information, especially if low numbers are present.*

*Children may be able to provide useful clean-catch urine specimens with the assistance of medical personnel or parents. Although "bagged" specimens from young children are available, suprapubic aspirates are the specimens of choice, with catheter specimens as a second choice.*

6. Stool specimens submitted for the recovery of acid-fast bacilli should be processed whether or not acid-fast bacteria are seen in the staining of an unprocessed specimen.

   *It is often difficult to recover acid-fast bacilli from fecal material because the heavy overgrowth with bowel flora cannot be prevented, and special procedures should be followed.*

   *Stool specimens from children infected with human immunodeficiency virus type 1 may be processed for acid-fast bacilli. Acid-fast stains are often positive in pediatric patients infected with* Mycobacterium avium-M. intracellulare.

7. Surface lesions (wounds) must be sampled carefully. It is imperative to open a surface lesion and sample the advancing margin of the lesion firmly. Purulent exudate must be expressed and aspirated or collected on swabs. Surface lesion samples are unsuitable for anaerobic studies.

   *Purulent exudate alone may not reveal growth on plating since the encased organisms may be dead. The representative specimen is from the advancing margin of the wound.*

   *Never submit a dry swab that has been carelessly rubbed over a surface lesion.*

   *Anaerobes are abundant on skin surfaces and are common surface wound contaminants; therefore, anaerobic cultures of surface wound samples are discouraged. Scrub the area around the wound carefully before sampling.*

   *In determining the agent of bacterial cellulitis, especially in children, the site can be anesthetized, a small volume of sterile, nonbacteriostatic saline injected into the subcutaneous area at the leading edge of the cellulitis, and the saline aspirated back into the syringe. The aspirate is then cultured.*

8. Wound specimens for anaerobic workup must be submitted in an appropriate anaerobic transport medium (Fig. 10).

   *Anaerobic transport media are designed to protect the strictest anaerobes. Other methods of transport may preserve some anaerobes for a time but may not allow their optimal recovery.*

   *The physician's need for complete anaerobic data underscores the laboratory's need for a specimen properly selected and submitted in an anaerobic transport medium.*

9. Nonspecific terms such as *"wound," "eye,"* and *"genital"* in the description of a specimen are not helpful to the laboratory. Use the names of the specific anatomic locations from which the specimen was taken.

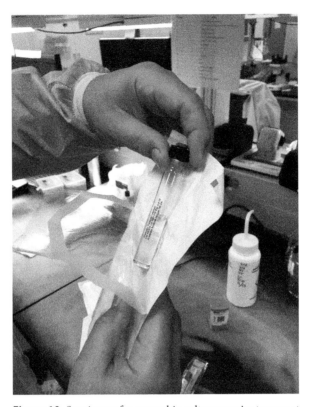

**Figure 10** Specimens for anaerobic culture require transport containers and conditions that protect the strictest anaerobes from exposure to oxygen. Many are available commercially for transport of swabs, tissues, and fluids, and manufacturer instructions should be followed where available.

10. Microbiology laboratories should have on hand the complete *Practical Guidance for Clinical Microbiology* (formerly *Cumitechs*) published by the American Society for Microbiology and the current editions of two or more helpful texts on clinical microbiology.

11. The American Society for Microbiology (21) and the Centers for Disease Control and Prevention (22) published recommendations for the collection of laboratory specimens associated with outbreaks of gastroenteritis. These recommendations cover specimen management for bacteria, viruses, and parasites associated with true or suspected outbreaks.

*A more recent publication for diagnosis and laboratory management of bacterial gastroenteritis may be helpful for health care and laboratory personnel reference (21).*

**12.** A recent document published in partnership between the American Society for Microbiology and the Infectious Diseases Society of America discusses specimen management from an anatomic system-based concept rather than by specimen types (23).

## Specimen Transport

**1.** It is critical that specimens for culture of all microbes be processed as soon as possible after collection, preferably within 1 to 2 h, and that the correct transport medium be used. If processing of urine samples will be delayed, they should be refrigerated, inoculated into primary isolation medium before transport, or transported in a preservative solution.

*Many species of bacteria are vulnerable to delays in processing, temperature changes, and decreased moisture; during prolonged transport, rapidly growing bacteria may overgrow more fastidious pathogens.*

*Because of the rapid generation time of many urinary tract pathogens (many bacteria can reproduce themselves every 20 to 30 min), colony counts for urine samples are invalid if the specimen is not processed within 30 min of receipt. If urine cannot be cultured within 30 min, refrigerate the specimen. Refrigerated transport or the use of an acceptable urine preservative is recommended if the specimen is to be sent by a private office to an external laboratory for processing.*

**2.** If a delay in transport is anticipated or if cultures for bacteria are to be sent to a reference laboratory, Stuart's, Amies, or Cary-Blair transport medium should be used. Dry swabs are unacceptable, although group A streptococci tend to survive well on dry swabs.

*Transport medium is formulated to maintain the viability of bacteria but allow only a slow rate of replication. However, fastidious strains may not survive in the nutritionally poor medium, and some bacterial populations may double within 1 h if body fluids are present.*

*Viral transport medium is necessary for all viral specimens collected by a swab. Aspirates, washings, tissues, and fluids for viral analysis can be submitted in sterile containers.*

*When a courier system is used for transport, several issues must be resolved, including the following: the amount of time that elapses between collection and pickup and arrival at the testing laboratory; the temperature in the courier vehicle and the need for temperature-controlled transport containers in the vehicle; the frequency of pickup; and the disposition of specimens arriving at the local laboratory after the final pickup of the day.*

*Transport conditions may differ for a clinical specimen and for a plated specimen.*

3. When possible, specimens should be delivered directly to the microbiology laboratory, bypassing central collection areas or other departments.

*We are not measuring chemicals, enzyme levels, or body cells, but measuring living, replicating organisms that cannot be expected to conform to our schedules of convenience no matter how busy we may be.*

## Specimen Processing: General

*Please include the correct source of the specimen. A significant problem we have in virology is that swabs arrive in the laboratory and their source is inappropriately labeled as "swab." Remember, the specimen source directs our decision of which cell types to use. A swab from a genital ulcer would be handled quite differently than one from the nasopharynx.*

KAREN CARROLL, M.D.
Johns Hopkins, Baltimore, MD

1. Specimens should not be processed until the laboratory requisition and label are correctly and completely prepared (Fig. 11). These items should provide antimicrobial therapy information about the patient, as well as the patient's working diagnosis, either in text or in *International Classification of Diseases* (ICD) code format.

*The person transcribing the physician's orders should be telephoned by the laboratory to complete the requisition or to verify questionable needs or responses.*

*Submitters should understand that the information requested is used by the laboratory to assist in laboratory interpretation of test results.*

2. Specimens should not be processed if they are received in inappropriate containers or improper transport medium or after a prolonged delay. Telephone the physician or nurse to determine whether a second specimen can be conveniently obtained.

*Insignificant, irrelevant, or incorrect information obtained from incorrectly collected or transported specimens may mislead the attending physician.*

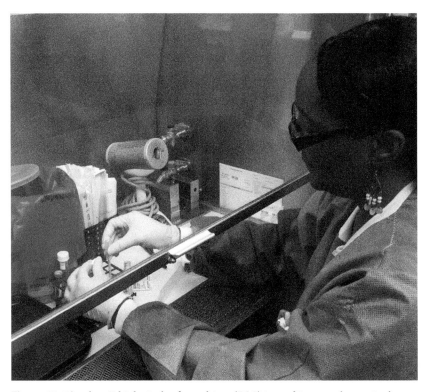

**Figure 11** The class II biological safety cabinet (BSC) is used in several areas in the laboratory. Here, the BSC is the required site for specimen opening and inoculation, and initial manipulations. Other BSCs will be used in the mycology and virology laboratory as well as for manipulation of *M. tuberculosis* specimens.

*Outpatient status or difficult collection procedures must be considered, and then an appropriate decision regarding a specific case can be made.*

*The final report should clearly indicate that the specimen was inadequate and that the results may or may not be valid or complete.*

3. A second specimen obtained from the same site within the same 24-h period should not be processed unless the physician has contacted the laboratory with justified specific orders to do so.

*Duplicate orders most commonly represent clerical errors, which are costly to the patient and take up unnecessary laboratory time. In only a few instances is processing of two cultures within 24 h clinically indicated.*

## Specimen Processing: Molecular

*We do not perform microbiological analysis that does not comply with acceptable practices. We do it right, or we don't do it!*

JAMES SNYDER, Ph.D.
University of Louisville, Louisville, KY

1. Presently, many of our infectious disease diagnostic procedures are conducted using genetic or proteomic approaches rather than, or in addition to, standard culture methods. In general, specimens for microbiological analysis are collected and transported to maintain the integrity and viability of the organism and not for any particular test method.

   *Molecular testing in the microbiology laboratory is no different from other test procedures in that the quality of the specimen submitted for analysis has a profound effect on the outcome of the test; tissues, fluids, washes, and aspirates are always preferred, and swab samples only when the suspected pathogen can be captured by swabbing (e.g., some viruses present in vesicles and* Chlamydia *in cervical columnar cells) or the preferred specimens cannot be obtained by any other means. Resist swab specimens that have been immersed in aspirated fluids and request the actual fluid for analysis.*

   *The majority of molecular microbiological assays are kit based and have usually been approved by the FDA for use in patient diagnostic testing. Manufacturers of FDA-cleared assays provide package inserts that often detail approved specimen types, recommended collection methods, and/or transport conditions.*

   *Manufacturer indications must be followed and, if a collection device is included, that device must be used. If the laboratory elects to change the device or a transport system of an FDA-cleared test kit, the new device must be fully validated by the laboratory before use.*

2. Nucleic acid amplification tests and PCR tests are sensitive enough to detect nucleic acid in almost any properly collected specimen (Fig. 12).

   *Follow the manufacturer's recommendations in the package insert.*

   *For laboratory-developed molecular tests, the collection device and the transport system must be validated in conjunction with performance of the assay itself.*

3. Matrix-assisted laser desorption ionization–time of flight mass spectrometry (MALDI-TOF MS) testing requires no special specimen management because this identification method is routinely used and FDA-cleared for identification of bacterial isolates from routine culture procedures.

*If direct specimen analysis is to be attempted with the MALDI-TOF instrument and it has not been FDA-cleared, the process must be validated prior to reporting results.*

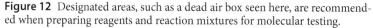

4. Multiplex and syndromic nucleic acid test instruments that are FDA-cleared provide manufacturer instructions for all approved tests, i.e., blood, gastrointestinal, and respiratory tract specimens, and these instructions should be followed unless the laboratory is going to validate the off-label use of specimens or collection devices.

**Figure 12**  Designated areas, such as a dead air box seen here, are recommended when preparing reagents and reaction mixtures for molecular testing.

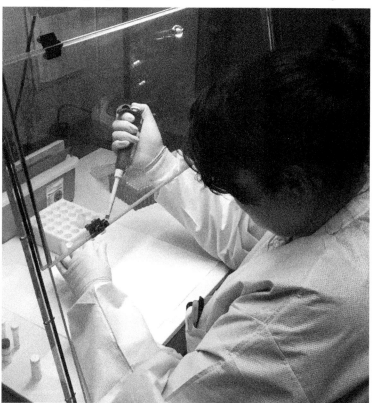

## Lower Respiratory Tract Specimens

1. Lower respiratory tract specimens include (in relative order of preference): BALs, bronchial brushings, bronchial washings, transbronchial lung biopsy specimens, and sputum.

   *Incorrectly labeled lower respiratory tract specimens could potentially result in errors and contribute to misdiagnosis and inappropriate therapy.*

   *BAL and bronchial washings are handled quite differently in the laboratory, so inappropriate labeling may affect culture interpretation.*

   *Because normal respiratory flora accompanies each of the above specimens, good laboratory practice dictates that the normal flora will be acknowledged but not worked up. Routine respiratory pathogens of concern will be:* Streptococcus pneumoniae, Staphylococcus aureus, Pseudomonas aeruginosa, Enterobacteriaceae, Haemophilus *sp.*, Moraxella catarrhalis, *and* Neisseria meningitidis. *Clearly, special requests may be honored.*

2. BAL specimens are the only respiratory specimens that can be quantitated, which requires a great deal of laboratory work and costs.

   *The BAL procedure washes cells from the airways (a <u>subsegmental bronchus: lingular</u>) that bronchoscopy cannot reach and necessitates in adults the installation of up to 100 ml of nonbacteriostatic saline in 20-ml increments (much less in children). This is the only specimen that should be labeled as a BAL.*

   *For reporting purposes, the laboratory will identify and do susceptibility tests on any two aerobic isolates. If three or more species are present (unless one is a frank pathogen), the interpretation becomes misleading and a descriptive, less definitive report will likely be issued.*

3. Bronchial washing is a poor predictor of the agents of pneumonia, and it is recommended that this specimen type is not submitted for that purpose.

   *To obtain a bronchial washing, the bronchoscope is generally wedged into a segmental bronchus. It requires only about 10 ml of nonbacteriostatic saline to be instilled and aspirated.*

   *Bronchial washings should not be mislabeled as a BAL. It is a bronchial washing and cannot be prepared for quantitative culture.*

   *For reporting purposes, the laboratory may identify and do susceptibility tests on any two aerobic isolates. Three or more isolates will be reported with a comment such as "Mixed respiratory flora. No predominant pathogen present."*

4. All routine sputum specimens should be evaluated by direct Gram stain to assess how representative of lower respiratory tract secretions they are. Some type of scoring system should be used.

   *Samples that are representative of oropharyngeal contamination (saliva) rather than true lower respiratory tract secretions produce insignificant results.*

   *The reporting of a potentially pathogenic bacterium in a nonrepresentative sputum sample can be misleading, particularly in cases of clinical pneumonitis.*

5. Only one sputum sample per 24 h should be submitted except for postbronchoscopy specimens. If more than one specimen is received in series, the first morning specimen or the one with no microscopic evidence of contamination should be selected for processing.

   *One sputum sample per 24 h is usually adequate to reflect the respiratory secretion pool.*

   *Postbronchoscopy specimens are usually the best deep-cough specimens that can be obtained.*

6. Sputum samples less than 2 ml in volume should not be processed unless the material is obviously purulent.

   *Small quantities of a clear, thin material (often with bubbles) usually represent saliva.*

   *With the exception of legionellosis, most respiratory bacterial infections cause copious amounts of sputum to be expectorated.*

7. Sputum specimens are rarely obtained in pediatric populations.

   *Respiratory tract infection is common in pediatric populations. A fundamental understanding of the anatomy of the respiratory tract and the associated flora is helpful in interpreting culture findings and providing clinically relevant information to the physician. For example, an adequate nasopharyngeal sample yields a specimen with ciliated columnar epithelial cells.*

   *Specimens acquired through the trachea are often contaminated with oropharyngeal flora, which may obscure identification of the true pathogen associated with a lower respiratory infection.*

   *In addition, children may be transiently colonized with nontypeable* H. influenzae, Streptococcus pneumoniae, *or* Neisseria meningitidis, *and care must be taken in the interpretation of cultures yielding these isolates.*

*In pediatric microbiology, children are not miniature adults!*

J. MICHAEL MILLER, Ph.D., (D)ABMM
Microbiology Technical Services, LLC,
Dunwoody, GA

8. Tracheal aspirates should be evaluated by Gram stain to determine the suitability of the specimen for culture (24).

   *Tracheal aspirates can be rejected for culture if a Gram stain reveals either "no organisms seen" or "≥10 squamous epithelial cells per low-power field."*

## Urine Specimens

1. Colony counts are routinely performed on all clean-catch urine specimens. For accurate culture interpretation, the requisition should indicate whether or not the patient is symptomatic for a urinary tract infection.

   *It is generally agreed that at least 100,000 CFU/ml of urine usually indicates a possible urinary tract infection in asymptomatic individuals. In symptomatic patients, counts of 10,000 or fewer may be significant. The significance of low-count urine samples is often validated by the presence of leukocytes in the specimen.*

   *In children, colony counts of a potential pathogen between 10,000 and 50,000 CFU/ml are usually regarded as significant. If the child is too young for successful collection of a clean-catch urine sample, procedures using suprapubic bladder aspiration, a temporary catheter, or a bag taped over the urogenital area for <30 min to collect urine are alternative techniques.*

2. Anaerobic cultures should not be set up for routine clean-catch urine.

   *Urinary tract infections are rarely caused by anaerobic bacteria. If an anaerobic infection is suspected, a suprapubic bladder aspiration should be performed.*

3. Material from Foley catheter tips should not be accepted for culture.

   *It is impossible to remove a urinary catheter without contaminating it with microorganisms inhabiting the urethra.*

4. Urine samples collected directly from indwelling catheter bags should not be accepted for culture. When specimens are to be taken from indwelling catheters, a needle and syringe should be used for urine aspiration through the sampling port after the port has been disinfected.

   *Stagnant urine in a catheter bag is overgrown with bacteria, making culture interpretation misleading and clinically irrelevant.*

   *More fastidious pathogens are also overgrown with more rapidly growing coliforms.*

   *Needleless sampling ports are now available on urinary catheters and offer a safer means of specimen collection.*

## Wound Specimens

*A real problem for many of us is receiving a specimen from a nonsterile source with inappropriate orders from the physician asking us to work up anything that grows.*
MARK LAROCCO, Ph.D., (D)ABMM
M.T.L. Consulting, Erie, PA

1. To determine whether wound samples represent superficial or deep specimens, direct Gram staining can be performed to evaluate the relative numbers of neutrophils and squamous epithelial cells (2).

   *Clinically infected wounds almost always produce a pyogenic reaction, and Gram stains should reveal many polymorphonuclear leukocytes.*

   *The presence of epithelial cells indicates a superficial sample or contamination from the skin of the wound margins. The laboratory may be reluctant to anaerobically culture wound (swab) specimens containing epithelial cells.*

   *A published scoring system of Gram stain evaluation of wound specimens is very helpful in determining the value of the specimen and the next steps to take in analysis (25).*

2. Anaerobic cultures should not be routinely set up for superficial-wound specimens or for specimens that have not been submitted in an appropriate anaerobic container.

   *Physicians should use clinical judgment when ordering anaerobic cultures. Preparation of these cultures is expensive and requires considerable technical expertise.*

   *Gas production, foul odor, and copious pus production are clinical indications of some anaerobic wound infections.*

3. Diagnosis of the bacterial etiology of pressure sores (decubiti) is notoriously difficult. Material from a swab is not the specimen of choice.

   *The specimen of choice is a tissue biopsy.*

   *Swab specimens from pressure sores tend to reflect surface colonization and may not allow detection of a true etiologic agent.*

   *Needle aspirates may result in underestimation of bacterial isolates compared with more accurate deep biopsy specimens.*

4. Used alone, the term "wound" is inadequate and usually inappropriate and should always be accompanied by the name of the specific anatomic site from which the sample was taken.

5. The specimen of choice is a sample from the advancing margin of the lesion, not the material and debris (pus) within the lesion.

*Surface wounds are notorious for containing contaminating and confusing commensal flora, especially if only a swab of the pus or debris covering the wound is submitted.*

*Surface wounds can be debrided using sponges moistened with sterile water or sterile nonbacteriostatic saline prior to firmly sampling the advancing margin of the lesion.*

*To prevent recontamination, a new sponge should be used with each wipe of the wound surface.*

*If a swab of the pus is submitted, a sample from the advancing margin should also be submitted on another swab.*

## Spinal Fluid Specimens

1.  Direct Gram stain evaluation should be performed on the cytocentrifuged sediments of all spinal fluids submitted for culture. All positive or negative results must be immediately telephoned to the physician.

    *Immediate results may represent lifesaving information in some cases of meningitis. Even a report of "no bacteria seen" is important information in the assessment of clinical cases.*

    *A simple stain (with methylene blue or crystal violet) or an acridine orange stain of spinal fluid also gives rapid information on the presence or absence of bacteria.*

2.  If specimen processing is to be delayed, spinal fluid should be placed in a 35°C incubator until it can be inoculated into culture medium. Spinal fluid should never be held in the refrigerator.

    *Spinal fluid (like urine) is a good culture medium. In most instances, infections are caused by one species, and overgrowth with contaminants is not a concern.*

    *Some organisms that cause meningitis are sensitive to chilling and may not survive refrigerator temperatures.*

3.  Direct antigen tests of spinal fluid may or may not provide accurate results and should be discouraged. Consider carefully the need for information from these antigen detection methods in the light of potential false-positive or false-negative results in a specific patient population.

    *Rarely is a direct antigen test of spinal fluid positive when a routine Gram stain is not also positive. In fact, false-positive results may occur with direct antigen tests in low-prevalence populations and may lead to a misdiagnosis and inappropriate therapy.*

## Throat and Nasopharyngeal Specimens

1. Throat specimens should be routinely processed for the recovery of beta-hemolytic streptococci only. While *Streptococcus pyogenes* is of primary concern because it can lead to sequelae, group C and group G beta-hemolytic streptococci can also be isolated from throat cultures of symptomatic patients. Additionally, *Arcanobacterium* (Gram-positive rod) and *Fusobacterium necrophorum* (anaerobe) may be important in some patients.

   *Organisms other than beta-hemolytic streptococci usually do not cause primary acute pharyngitis. Staphylococci may cause tonsillar abscesses,* H. influenzae *causes constrictive epiglottitis, and* Corynebacterium diphtheriae *causes membranous pharyngitis.*

   *If* Neisseria gonorrhoeae *or another non-beta-hemolytic streptococcus is suspected, the laboratory must be notified.*

   *Direct methods designed to detect the antigen of group A streptococci lack sensitivity in cases where low numbers of organisms may be present on the membranes or where an improper specimen collection technique has been used. Negative antigen tests still require culture or DNA probe confirmation in children but may not be needed in adult patients (23).*

2. Attempts to recover *H. influenzae* from routine throat cultures are the prerogative of each hospital or laboratory but should be discouraged, even in children.

   *A high percentage of healthy adults and children harbor* Haemophilus *spp. in their oropharynx.*

   *Physicians must inform the laboratory if a* Haemophilus *sp. is suspected.*

   *Epiglottitis is best confirmed by a blood culture, never a throat culture. Using a swab can induce spasms of the inflamed epiglottis. Because of the widespread use of conjugated* Haemophilus *vaccines in children, epiglottitis and meningitis due to* H. influenzae *are now rare.*

3. Antimicrobial susceptibility tests should not be performed on bacterial isolates from throat cultures unless the patient is allergic to penicillins.

   *Beta-hemolytic streptococci (particularly group A streptococci) remain universally susceptible to penicillin.*

   *Other organisms are not considered a cause of acute pharyngitis in the absence of specific complications. The decision to treat other causes of bacterial pharyngitis is left to the physician; however, susceptibility testing is not required because of the wide variety of agents that can be used to treat such infections.*

4. Coliform bacilli in throat cultures are not usually reported.

   *Coliform bacilli do not normally cause pharyngitis but can colonize the throat and serve as a reservoir for lower respiratory tract infections.*

   *Hospitalized patients tend to be colonized with coliform organisms that are resistant to many antibiotics used in the hospital.*

   *Susceptibility tests should not be performed except on request or for infection control purposes.*

5. Sinusitis can be diagnosed clinically with no specimen for culture. The appropriate specimen for culture is a needle aspirate from the infected sinus, not material from a swab.

   *The microbiology of sinusitis is well known, and empiric therapy is usually the therapy of choice.*

   *Results from throat, nasal drainage, or routine nasopharyngeal cultures usually do not correlate well with the true etiologic agent of sinus infection. Therefore, a needle aspirate from the sinus is the specimen of choice.*

6. Careful attention to throat specimen collection for direct antigen tests is just as important as the type of specimen taken for culture.

   *All direct antigen tests for group A streptococcus in the throat have limited ability to detect the organism. It is recommended that negative direct antigen tests be followed by culture. Poorly collected throat samples may have a limited number of group A streptococci on the swab, thereby causing the direct antigen test to exhibit weakly positive or negative results.*

## Vaginal and Endometrial Specimens

*As more of our testing becomes available by molecular methods, clinicians and laboratorians need to learn when to probe, when to amplify, and when to culture.*

LISA L. STEED, Ph.D.
Medical University of South Carolina,
Charleston, SC

1. In general, vaginal cultures are of minimal value, and laboratories should resist processing them. Specimens for *N. gonorrhoeae* culture should be obtained directly from the uterine cervix. Anaerobic culture should not be performed except on abscess fluid aspirated by syringe and needle from a perivaginal abscess. Other infections and syndromes, such as trichomoniasis, candidiasis, and bacterial vaginosis can be diagnosed by direct mounts, Gram-stained smears, PCR, and other tests.

*The normal vaginal flora includes a wide variety of aerobic and anaerobic organisms. Anaerobic cultures of vaginal swab specimens are impossible to interpret in light of the normal background flora (Fig. 13).*

*Direct Gram staining of vaginal secretions in a search for* N. gonorrhoeae *may be misleading because of the various resident organisms that can morphologically mimic* N. gonorrhoeae-*like organisms.*

*Physicians should be discouraged from submitting vaginal swab specimens for culture to diagnose bacterial vaginosis. Gram stain evaluation should be used to document the change in commensal flora, and is discussed in Cumitech 17A (26).*

2. Endometrial samples should be collected with a protected suction curette and placed in an anaerobic transport container. These specimens should always be processed for aerobic and anaerobic organisms.

*Because the environment of the endometrial cavity is relatively anaerobic, anaerobic infections are not uncommon.*

*In cases of postpartum infection, organisms such as group B streptococci and* Listeria monocytogenes *should be specifically cultured. A double-lumen catheter should be used to collect the specimen.*

3. Vaginal specimens (26) from prepubescent girls can be cultured to determine the etiologic agent of premenarchal vulvovaginitis or a sexually transmitted disease.

*Several factors contribute to the development of vulvovaginitis in girls (i): anatomic differences in the immature vagina (ii), a neutral pH that encourages bacterial overgrowth, and (iii) a lack of good hygiene, resulting in fecal contamination of the vulvar and urethral areas.*

*Most sexually transmitted diseases in prepubertal girls cause vaginitis rather than cervicitis. A sample of any discharge that is present can be appropriately submitted for bacterial culture.*

*For children with minimal discharge, an intravaginal specimen is required.* Gonorrhea, Chlamydia, *and general vaginal cultures are prepared in accordance with laboratory protocol. Rapid antigen detection or immunofluorescence assays for detection of gonococci or chlamydiae are contraindicated for use in testing specimens collected from a prepubertal child.*

*Any vesicles noted should be sampled for herpes simplex virus culture.*

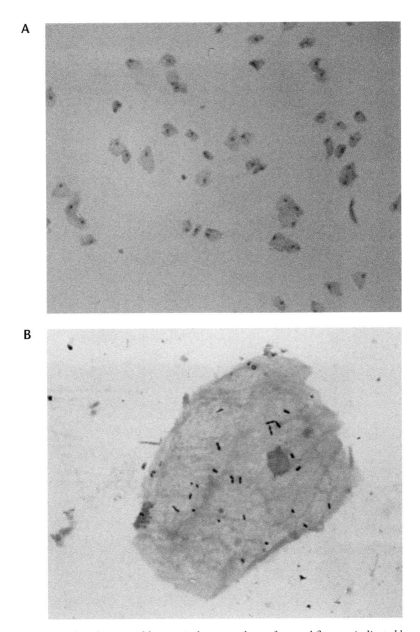

**Figure 13** Vaginal swabs invariably contain large numbers of normal flora, as indicated by the presence of large numbers of epithelial cells seen first at low power (A) and then under oil immersion (B). Interpretation is difficult.

## Miscellaneous Specimens

1. In processing eye cultures, enriched chocolate agar should be used to detect fastidious organisms such as *Haemophilus* spp., *Neisseria* spp., or slow-growing Gram-negative bacilli. A direct Gram stain should always be examined at the time cultures are set up.

   *Fastidious organisms often infect the eye and may be overlooked if an enriched culture medium is not used.*

   *The presence of Gram-negative bacilli that morphologically resemble* Pseudomonas *spp. should immediately be made known to the physician because these organisms can rapidly cause blinding ophthalmitis.*

2. Tissue biopsy specimens for bacterial or viral culture, but not fungal culture, should be processed only after being homogenized with a stomacher or minced and ground with a sterile pestle and mortar.

   *Anaerobic cultures should be set up on request or if gas or a foul odor is detected by the physician or technologist. Anaerobic cultures may be valid only if the tissue has been submitted in a container protected from exposure to atmospheric oxygen, although in larger specimens the reducing properties of the tissue proteins tend to maintain a relative anaerobic environment.*

   *Tissue imprint smears followed by direct Gram staining of the ground eluate should be performed, and any positive findings should be reported immediately to the physician.* Clostridium perfringens *can be immediately detected by Gram staining. Other organisms, such as staphylococci and streptococci, also have characteristic morphologies.*

   *Fungal hyphae may be disrupted during homogenization; therefore, a piece of the tissue should be planted onto media for mycology workup.*

3. Gastric specimens in general do not yield meaningful culture results except perhaps for septic infants or for older individuals with obstructions high in the intestine. Bacterial colony counts for gastric secretions are of questionable value and should be discouraged.

   *Anaerobic bacteria can inhabit normal gastric secretions, and interpretations of culture results may be difficult.*

   *The presence of large numbers of bacteria in gastric secretions usually indicates an alkaline pH shift caused by regurgitation of duodenal secretions in patients with intestinal obstructions.*

   *The recovery of certain species of mycobacteria may be significant. Gastric aspirates for mycobacteria should be neutralized before they are held for processing.*

4. Do not hesitate to ask for or recommend an Infectious Disease consult when complicated specimen issues arise.

# Specimen Collection and Processing

*This section serves two purposes:*
*1. To assist medical staff in the details of selection, collection, and transport of clinical specimens for microbiologic analysis, and*
*2. To provide a model for use in writing the specimen management portion of the laboratory procedures manual.*

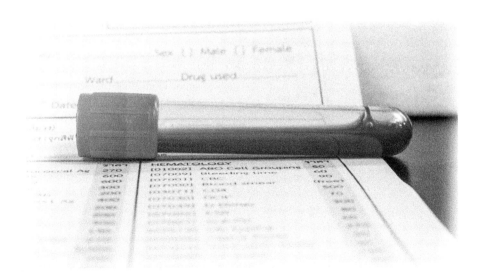

*There once was a surgeon named Peters*
*Who drained from an abscess three liters,*
*But sent only a swab*
*Labeled "Thing-a-ma-bob"*
*For five cultures, six stains, and two titers.*
*(Hint: Proper quantity and site make cultures turn out right.)*

JILL E. CLARRIDGE III, Ph.D., ABMM
Seattle, Washington

# BODY FLUID SPECIMENS

## ■ Abdominal-Peritoneal Fluid (Paracentesis, Ascites)

**A.** Selection
   1. Aspirate the specimen of choice from the peritoneal cavity.
   2. The patient usually has a distended abdomen, weight gain, and a decrease in urinary output.

**B.** Collection
   1. Materials (disposable kits are available)
      a. Trocar and cannula or dialysis catheter and a long needle
      b. Scalpel
      c. Skin disinfectant
      d. Local anesthetic
      e. Sterile specimen container
      f. Suture set
   2. Method
      a. Prepare the skin site for puncture or incision. The patient should be in a sitting position.
      b. The surgeon punctures the skin 3 to 5 cm below the umbilicus in the midline and introduces a dialysis catheter into the pouch of Douglas. The procedure can be guided by ultrasound.
      c. When aspiration reveals gross blood or intestinal contents, a laparotomy is performed; if not, washings are done with 1 liter of saline or balanced salt solution.
      d. If allowed to drain normally, the fluid is often thick and flows very slowly. Several hundred milliliters may be drained.

**C.** Labeling
   1. Label the specimen with patient information.
   2. Include the time of collection and all diagnostic information.

**D.** Transport
   1. Do *not* refrigerate the specimen.
   2. Transport the specimen directly to the laboratory.

**E.** Comment: See Table 10.
   Pediatric needs: Same as for adults.

**Table 10** Specimen management of sterile body fluids[a]

| Fluid | Collection container | Concentration | Stain | Comment[b] |
|---|---|---|---|---|
| Amniotic | Anaerobe tube | No | Gram stain | |
| Culdocentesis | Anaerobe tube | No | Gram stain | |
| Dialysis effluent | Isolator or sterile tube or urine cup or two blood culture bottles | Centrifuge or filter | Gram stain or acridine orange stain | Low detection rate by staining. <100 WBCs/ml is normal. Use one-third of filter on each of three media. |
| Peritoneal (ascites) | 10 ml in each of two blood culture bottles plus an anaerobe tube | Cytocentrifuge from tube | Gram stain from cytocentrifuge | <300 WBCs/ml is normal. |
| Pleural (effusion, transudate, thoracentesis, empyema) | Anaerobe tube | Cytocentrifuge from tube | Gram stain from cytocentrifuge | >5 ml needed for fungi. No WBCs or a few WBCs are normal. Empyema has many WBCs. |
| Synovial | Blood culture bottle plus anaerobe tube | Cytocentrifuge from tube | Gram stain from cytocentrifuge | A few WBCs are normal. |

[a]Adapted from reference 41.
[b]WBC, white blood cell. Any cytocentrifuged sediment can be cultured or stained.

## ◼ Blood Specimens

New information on blood culture procedures continues to emerge. Frequent literature review is recommended.

*If I had one thing to tell medical students, it would be to always submit two separate blood collections for "blood culture."*

PAUL SOUTHERN, Ph.D., ABMM
University of Texas Southwestern Medical Center,
Dallas, TX

A. Selection (Practice universal precautions.)
   1. For the selection protocol, see Table 11.
   2. The method of specimen collection and the amount of blood drawn directly influence the success of recovery of isolates and the interpretation of results. Alter this procedure according to the protocols used at your own institution. Refer to Cumitech 1C (27).
   3. Factors directly influencing culture results:
      a. Volume of blood collected: perhaps most important
      b. Method of skin disinfection: critical
         The number of temporally spaced cultures and the timing of collections may not be as critical as once thought, but may be important in specific clinical situations.
   4. Collection of blood through a peripheral or indwelling central venous catheter is often fraught with error because of contamination by commensal flora. Culture results for blood from catheter collection need accompanying results for a venous-collected specimen to aid in interpretation. See pediatric needs comment below.

B. Collection
   1. Materials
      a. Sterile gloves
      b. Alcohol and tincture of iodine
      c. Double-needle collection set
      d. Aerobic *and* anaerobic blood culture bottles. Pediatric bottles may also be available. See Comments.
      e. Tourniquet
   2. Method
      a. Remove the outer seal and cap from each blood culture bottle and swab the rubber stopper with a sterile alcohol preparation. Allow the alcohol to dry.
      b. Clamp the tubing with the hemostat and insert one needle into the aerobic bottle.

**Table 11** Conditions and protocols for collecting blood specimens

| Clinical condition | Protocol | Comment |
|---|---|---|
| Adults and adolescents Severe septicemia, meningitis, osteomyelitis, arthritis, pneumonia | Two cultures before therapy | One 10- to 20-ml sample from each arm |
| Subacute bacterial endocarditis | Three cultures in 24 h | Space collection over 24 h. Collect two at start of fever spikes. Collect three more if the first two are negative after 24 h. |
| Acute bacterial endocarditis | Three cultures within 1 to 2 h before therapy | |
| Low-grade intravascular infection | Three cultures in 24 h | Space collections at least 1 h apart. Collect two at first sign of febrile episode. |
| Bacteremia of unknown origin (patient on therapy) | Four to six cultures in 48 h | Collect specimen just before administration of antibiotic. |
| Younger children | 1- to 2-ml samples | Two cultures are usually adequate for diagnosing bacteremia in newborns. |

    c. Prepare the skin for venipuncture.
       i. Palpate for a vein to locate the venipuncture site. Decontaminate the skin site with a commercial product such as chlorhexidine, or follow steps ii and iii below.
      ii. Beginning in the center of the area and moving outward in concentric circles, swab the site with alcohol.
     iii. Swab the site with an iodophor in the same manner. Allow the iodine to remain for 30 s to 1 min.
     iv. Optional: Remove residual iodine with another alcohol swab.

*For adults*
      v. Without repalpating for the vein, perform the venipuncture with the other end of the double-needle set.
     vi. Remove the hemostat and allow blood to flow into the bottle (5 ml into a 50-ml bottle, 10 ml into a 100-ml bottle). Manufacturers of blood culture instruments may have different protocols. Follow them and always ensure the proper amount of blood is drawn into each bottle.
    vii. Clamp the hemostat and move the needle from the aerobic bottle to the anaerobic bottle. *Changing the needle before inoculating the second bottle creates a risk of contamination.*
   viii. Release the hemostat and allow blood to flow into the anaerobic bottle.

ix. Reclamp the hemostat.
x. As the needle is removed from the patient's arm, apply pressure with a gauze pad, and ask the patient to hold the pad tightly in place for 2 to 3 min.
xi. Remove the needle from the anaerobic bottle, and discard the collection set. *Do not recap the needles.*
xii. Label the bottles carefully.

*For children*
xiii. Draw blood (0.5 to 2 ml) from children with a needle and syringe and aspirate the blood into blood bottles prepared as described above.
xiv. Clean any blood from the top and sides of the bottle.

C. Labeling
   1. Label the specimen with patient information.
   2. Indicate the time of collection and the site (e.g., left arm).
   3. Note whether the patient is on antibiotics.
   4. Include the suspected diagnosis.

D. Transport
   1. Do *not* refrigerate the specimen. Hold it at room temperature or 35°C.
   2. Transport the specimen to the laboratory quickly. Organisms will continue to metabolize during holding and transport so the bottle must be placed on the instrument as soon after the draw as possible.

E. Comments
   New data suggest that anaerobic blood bottles may not be necessary for obtaining accurate and clinically relevant results. Two aerobic bottles may be more valuable because of the increase in the volume of blood cultured. A total of 20 to 30 ml of blood may be optimal. In addition, information obtained from a bottle or from a method for fungal (yeast) isolation may be more valuable than that obtained from the anaerobe bottle.
   1. Ideally, collect blood during the hour before a predicted fever spike or as the spike begins.
   2. Collect blood just before the administration of antibiotics.
   3. If possible, draw two sets at the same time. One from the right arm and one from the left. Volume of blood is more important than timing.
   4. A *total* of three cultures per 24 h is usually sufficient to rule out bacteremia or endocarditis. A sample for culture is a draw of at least 10 ml of blood divided between two bottles. Larger volumes may be more productive.
   5. Blood for culture should not be withdrawn through an indwelling intravenous or intra-arterial catheter unless it cannot be obtained by venipuncture. The problem lies in contamination of the catheter, not of the blood for culture. If possible, draw blood below an existing intravenous line to prevent dilution of the blood with infusion fluid.

6. Bone specimens
   a. Place the bone fragment in liquid medium.
   b. Transport the specimen rapidly.
   c. Each specimen must be accompanied by a smear from the culture site *and* a blood culture. This allows a more accurate interpretation of results.
   d. Patient information is important.
7. Bone marrow
   a. Inoculate a blood culture bottle (or agar medium if the specimen volume is small). Contact the laboratory (a lysis centrifugation method may be preferred).
   b. Ensure aseptic technique.
   c. The requisition should indicate the suspected diagnosis.
8. Indwelling central venous catheter: After disinfection, the connection between the extension tubing or cap and the hub is disconnected. The hub is then also disinfected. A sterile syringe is attached, and a minimum of 0.5 to 1.0 ml of blood is withdrawn and discarded in order to eliminate any interfering factors or contaminants from the line prior to collection of the blood for culture. A second sterile syringe is then attached, and an additional volume of 0.5 ml is withdrawn for culture. After disinfection of the septum of the collection bottle, the blood is inoculated into the bottle. The catheter is then flushed with heparin or saline.
9. Pediatric needs: The collection of blood culture specimens from children is often impeded by the reluctance of the child to cooperate during collections and the lack of easily accessible veins. In addition, collection of the specimen volumes recommended for adults is not possible with children. Although 0.5 ml is recommended as a minimum collection volume in children, in certain circumstances as little as 0.1 ml may be inoculated into a pediatric blood culture bottle. This small volume is usually adequate for only one bottle. Because of these factors, skin preparation is critical and disinfectants are allowed to dry for 1 min prior to venipuncture. In this population an anaerobic bottle is usually not necessary unless the patient is at risk for anaerobic septicemia.

---

*Regarding skin preparation with iodine for venipuncture: Bacteria are killed by drying, not by drowning.*

FRANK KOONTZ, Ph.D.
University of Iowa Hospitals, Iowa City, IA

## ▨ Cerebrospinal Fluid

**A.** Selection
  1. Collect the specimen using strict aseptic technique.
  2. The patient should be fasting.
  3. When only one tube of fluid is available, the microbiology laboratory receives it first. If more than one tube (1 ml each) is available, microbiology should receive the second or third tube, whichever is less bloody.
  4. Draw CSF at L3 to L4 or lower to avoid spinal cord damage. Draw it at L4 to L5 in children because the conus medullaris extends lower in children than in adults.

**B.** Collection
  1. Materials
     a. CSF tray
     b. Skin disinfectant
     c. Sterile towels or drape
     d. Novocaine (0.5 to 1%), needle, syringe
     e. Two lumbar puncture needles, small bore (20 to 22 gauge) with stylet
     f. Water manometer
     g. Three small sterile screw-cap tubes
  2. Method
     a. Ensure that the patient is motionless during the procedure. Restraints may be necessary.
     b. Explain that some pain is inevitable. Local anesthesia rarely reaches the meninges, and pain occurs when the needle stretches the dura and pulls on connective tissue around the vertebrae.
     c. Have the patient arch his or her back so that the head almost touches the knees.
     d. Disinfect the skin along a line drawn between the crests of the two ilia if a puncture is to be made in the lumbar region.
     e. The physician introduces the needle. A stylet is used to avoid implantation of skin, which may cause dermoid cysts to form in the spinal canal.
     f. As soon as the fluid starts to drop from the needle, the needle's position in the subarachnoid space is established.
     g. Measure the pressure of the CSF at this point.
     h. Collect the drops of fluid (as much as 1 ml if possible) in sterile screw-cap tubes.

**C.** Labeling
  1. Label the specimen with patient information.
  2. Indicate the age of the patient on the requisition.
  3. Indicate any therapy being given.

**D.** Transport
1. Do *not* refrigerate the specimen.
2. Hand-carry the specimen to the laboratory immediately.

**E.** Comments
1. Cytocentrifuge the fluid and evaluate the fluid by Gram stain, read the results within 30 min to 1 h if possible, and telephone the results to the physician.
2. It is essential that any culture and stain information about the CSF be telephoned or given to the physician immediately so that therapy can be evaluated early.
3. The age of the patient is a clue to the technologist as to the possible agent causing the illness.
4. Pediatric needs
   a. Collection of CSF may be more common in pediatric populations in order to rule out possible central nervous system infection whose symptoms may not be exhibited as expected. Performing a lumbar puncture is more difficult with pediatric patients because of problems involving positioning and restraint of the patient during the procedure, as well as limitations in the amount of fluid that can be collected from younger children and infants. As with adults, a traumatic tap is indicated by the presence of blood in the fluid specimen. If the puncture has been successful, the blood will cease to be present as more fluid is collected; however, if a grossly bloody or clotted specimen is obtained, the tap should be repeated since this may indicate incorrect placement of the needle during the procedure. Unfortunately, an immediate repeat tap in a sick child may not be possible, and it is often necessary to forward the bloody CSF to the laboratory for culture. The clot must be homogenized in the laboratory before culture.
   b. Certain pediatric populations are fitted with various types of ventricular shunts for drainage of excess CSF. It is important to label these specimens "ventricular shunt fluid" and *not* "CSF." Isolates that could be considered contaminants if obtained from a lumbar puncture may be serious pathogens in ventricular shunt infections.

### ▨ Pleural-Thoracentesis Fluid

**A.** Selection
   1. Fluid accumulation can cause pain, dyspnea, and other symptoms of pressure. Transudative effusions may issue from the heart (congestive heart failure) or kidneys or may be the result of vascular disease; exudative effusions are associated with inflammatory conditions such as parapneumonia and tuberculous empyema. Fluid can also be associated with lung infections.
   2. An aspirate of 10 ml of chest fluid is optimum.
   3. Collect the specimen by needle aspiration. Submit the fluid to microbiology, not a swab dipped into the fluid.

**B.** Collection
   1. Materials (Disposable kits are available.)
      a. Sterile drapes
      b. Skin disinfectant
      c. Novocaine (0.5 or 1%), needle, syringe
      d. Aspirating set (vacuum bottle)
      e. Mechanical or manual suction device
      f. Different-bore needles (small for serous fluid, large for purulent exudate)
      g. Optional: plastic catheter, hollow-bore needle (e.g., size 14 angiocatheter)
   2. Method
      a. Have the patient lie on his or her side in a semirecumbent position with the arm held above the head or forward. Alternatively, pillows can be used to support the upper body, and the patient can lean forward from a sitting position or can lean on the bedside table.
      b. Fluid collects in the interior and costophrenic sinus (where the lungs do not fill the pleural space).
      c. Disinfect the skin at the puncture site selected by the physician. Use an X ray and percussion (chest sounds) to help locate the site.
      d. Anesthetize the puncture site.
      e. Insert the needle between the ribs during inspiration to avoid the intercostal blood vessels lying along the inferior margins of the ribs.
      f. Do not allow the patient to cough.
      g. Prevent air from entering the cavity by placing a three-way stopcock on the needle.
      h. Attach the syringe or tubing from the vacuum bottle to the needle.
      i. On the physician's direction, open the stopcock and drain the fluid.

    j. Place the material for culture directly into a small sterile screw-cap jar.

    k. Place exudative (high protein) fluid in a lavender-top tube for a more accurate cell count and differential (Table 2).

**C.** Labeling

    1. Label the specimen with patient information.

    2. On the label, note the specific type of fluid and what studies are to be done.

**D.** Transport

    1. Transport the specimen directly to the laboratory.

    2. Do *not* refrigerate the specimen.

**E.** Comments

    1. A suction apparatus is necessary because fluid does not flow out by gravity. The low pressure is due to the elasticity of lung tissue and the resistance this tissue offers to the elevated ribs and lung expansion. The downward pull of the lung makes the pressure in the thoracic cavity lower than the atmospheric pressure outside the body.

    2. Observe sputum for the presence of blood, which suggests injury to lung tissue.

    3. Pediatric needs: Same as for adults.

# GASTROINTESTINAL SPECIMENS

## ▨ Duodenal Contents

**A.** Selection
1. The specimen of choice for demonstrating *Giardia lamblia* is a fecal specimen. The stool specimen may be nonproductive, however, and when symptoms persist, other means may be necessary to demonstrate the organism.
2. The duodenum is often the location of infections due to *G. lamblia* and *Strongyloides stercoralis.*
3. Two methods can be used for collecting duodenal material for analysis: intubation for duodenal aspiration or a swallowed duodenal capsule technique called Entero-Test.

**B.** Collection
1. Intubation (15-min procedure)
   a. Materials
      i. Double-lumen Diamond tube with the insertion length premeasured
      ii. Sedative (pentobarbital or other)
      iii. Syringe for aspiration or mechanical suction device
      iv. Large sterile screw-cap tube for specimen
   b. Method
      i. Following an overnight fast, administer a sedative parenterally.
      ii. Insert the double-lumen Diamond tube into the mouth and pass it 45 cm to the cardia.
      iii. Place the patient in the left lateral decubitus position with the head raised about 40.5 cm. Then have the patient swallow the tube another 15 cm to the greater curvature of the stomach.
      iv. The patient sits on the edge of the table with the body bent forward to assist entrance of the tube into the antrum.
      v. The patient lies in the right lateral decubitus position with the feet elevated for 5 min to allow peristalsis to move the tube into the duodenum.
      vi. Finally, the patient lies on his or her back for 5 min while the tube is slowly advanced 10 to 15 cm.
      vii. Adjust the final destination by fluoroscopy.

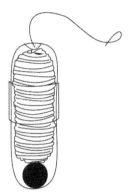

**Figure 14**  Drawing of an Entero-Test capsule. In comparison with intubation, this capsule allows a less invasive examination of duodenum contents for parasitic infection.

2. Capsule (Entero-Test) (28)
   a. Materials
      i.   The Entero-Test consists of a gelatin capsule containing a weighted, coiled length of nylon yarn or string. The end of the string or yarn protrudes through the top of the capsule (Fig. 14).
   b. Methods
      i.   Tape the protruding string to the patient's face.
      ii.  When the patient swallows the capsule, the gelatin dissolves and the weighted string is carried by peristalsis into the duodenum.
      iii. After 4 h, the string is recovered through the oral cavity, and the string portion, containing bile mucus, is sent to the laboratory.

C. Labeling
   1. Label the specimen with patient information.
   2. For the Entero-Test, indicate the length of time the capsule string was in the duodenum.
   3. Indicate the suspected diagnosis.

D. Transport
   1. For the Entero-Test, the string must arrive at the laboratory promptly to prevent drying. Hand-carry it, and preserve it in formalin if it will not be examined within 1 h.
   2. Duodenal drainage from intubation should be submitted unpreserved. If it will not be completely examined within 2 h, preserve it in formalin.
   3. Do *not* refrigerate the specimen.

E. Comments
   1. Immediate laboratory examination of the contents or string by direct mount or emulsion in 1 ml of saline is imperative.
   2. Do *not* allow the string to dry out.
   3. Check the pH and color of the terminal end of the string to document adequate passage into the duodenum.
   4. See Table 12 for appropriate preservatives for parasitology specimens.
   5. Pediatric needs: For a gastric aspirate, the contents are aspirated and placed in a sterile container for immediate transfer to the laboratory. Neutralization of the specimen must occur on arrival at the laboratory. Although an early morning fasting specimen is preferred for mycobacterial culture, infants on feeding schedules may not be able to provide such a sample. Medical and nursing staff should be encouraged to collect the aspirate as long after the last feeding as possible. If formula or other such food products are present in the aspirate, care must be taken in the interpretation of culture results if a mycobacterial species other than *Mycobacterium tuberculosis* is isolated.

**Table 12** Characteristics of preservatives used to transport feces for parasite examination[a]

| Preservative[b] | Used for concentrating sample? | Used with permanent stain? | Used with immunoassays? | Compatible with NATs? | Good fixative? | Contains mercury? | Problems with morphologies on staining? |
|---|---|---|---|---|---|---|---|
| Formalin[d] | ✓ | | ✓ | (✓)[e] | ✓ | | ✓ |
| Buffered formalin | ✓ | | ✓ | | ✓ | | ✓ |
| MIF | ✓ | (✓)[f] | | | | | ✓ |
| SAF[g] | ✓ | ✓[h] | ✓ | | ✓ | | |
| PVA | ✓[i] | ✓ | | (✓)[e] | ✓ | ✓ | ✓[i] |
| Modified PVA[j] | ✓ | ✓ | | ✓ | ✓ | ✓ | ✓ |
| Schaudin's fluid (no PVA)[j] | | ✓ | | ✓ | ✓ | ✓ | |
| Single-vial formulations[k] | ✓ | ✓ | ✓ | ✓ | ✓ | | ✓ |

[a]Data from reference 28 and reviewed in reference 42.
[b]MIF, merthiolate-iodine-formalin; SAF, sodium acetate-acetic acid-formalin; PVA, polyvinyl alcohol.
[c]Nucleic acid test; check manufacturer's recommendations.
[d]Formalin (5 or 10%) is often selected by manufacturers as an all-purpose fixative.
[e]Generally poor performance unless specified by the manufacturer.
[f]The iodine in MIF allows observation of protozoa (cysts), eggs, and larvae without further staining.
[g]A good choice if a single preservative is preferred, but albumin-coated slides are required.
[h]Iron hematoxylin stain provides a better view of organism morphology.
[i]Trichuris eggs and giardia cysts are not concentrated as easily as from formalin. Isospora oocysts may not be seen. Strongyloides larval morphology is poor.
[j]Many of these fixatives use a zinc sulfate base rather than a mercuric chloride base.
[k]Contains no mercury, formalin, or PVA.

## ▪ Gastric Contents

A. Selection
1. This method is used to examine for *M. tuberculosis* when sputum specimens are unavailable.
2. The method is often used with children younger than 7 years old.
3. Culture of gastric aspirates of newborns is not recommended routinely because misleading information may result (29).
4. Collect the specimen in the early morning before food and water intake.

B. Collection
1. Materials
   a. No. 14 or no. 16 Levin tube (for nasal insertion)
   b. Rehfuss or similar tube (for oral insertion)
   c. Local anesthetic spray (optional)
   d. Syringe or mechanical suction device
   e. Sterile specimen container
2. Method
   a. The patient should be sitting or lying on the left side with the head elevated 45°.
   b. With the patient's chin elevated, direct the Levin tube slightly upward and then gently push it posteriorly into the nasopharynx and esophagus.
   c. The nasopharynx may or may not be sprayed with a local anesthetic.
   d. For oral intubation, the tube can be chilled with ice to reduce nausea.
   e. Instruct the patient to open the mouth and project the chin forward and upward.
   f. Place the tip of the tube on the back of the tongue, avoiding the uvula, and push it into the posterior pharynx.
   g. Encourage the patient to close the mouth and alternate swallowing and deep oral breathing while the tube is pushed intermittently during swallowing to its destination, about 55 cm from the mouth.
   h. Use fluoroscopy to guide the tip into the antrum (if the patient is sitting) or into the middle of the greater curvature (if the patient is lying on the left side) (Fig. 15).
   i. Aspiration is accomplished by syringe or by mechanical means.

C. Labeling
1. Label the specimen with patient information.
2. Indicate the age of the patient and the suspected pathogen.
3. Note the time of collection.

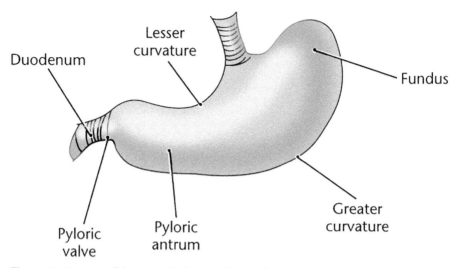

**Figure 15**  Diagram of the stomach, showing the antral region.

**D.** Transport
  1. Transport the specimen to the laboratory quickly.
  2. Refrigerate the specimen if transport will be delayed.

**E.** Comment: When sputum induction is followed in 30 min by gastric lavage, the combined specimens often yield more positive cultures for *M. tuberculosis* than sputum or gastric lavage alone.

## Pinworm Eggs Collected by Adhesive Tape Preparation

**A.** Selection
  1. Pinworms (*Enterobius vermicularis*) migrate through the rectum and deposit their eggs on the perianal skin, that is, on and around the anus.
  2. The worms usually lay their eggs periodically at night while the patient sleeps.
  3. The best specimens are obtained in the early morning before bathing.

**B.** Collection
  1. Materials. Special commercially available specimen collection paddles are preferred (Fig. 16). If they are unavailable, use the method below (Fig. 17).
     a. A piece of 2- to 2.5-cm-wide clear cellulose (Scotch) tape (not the invisible kind)
     b. Microscope slide (ca. 2.5 × 7.5 cm)
     c. Tongue depressor

**Figure 16** Plastic collection device for obtaining specimen for pinworm analysis.

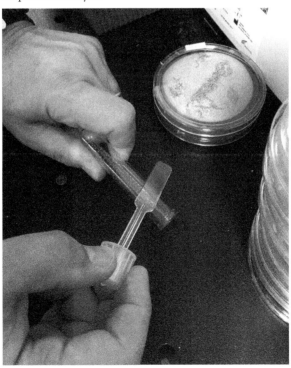

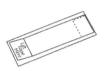

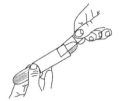

**A** Cellulose tape slide preparation

**B** Hold slide against tongue depressor one inch from end and lift long portion of tape from slide

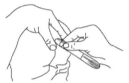

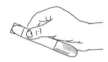

**C** Loop tape over end of depressor to expose gummed surface

**D** Hold tape and slide against tongue depressor

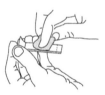

**E** Press gummed surfaces against several areas of perianal region

**F** Replace tape on slide

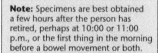

**G** Smooth tape with cotton or gauze

**Note:** Specimens are best obtained a few hours after the person has retired, perhaps at 10:00 or 11:00 p.m., or the first thing in the morning before a bowel movement or both.

**Figure 17** Alternative method for pinworm collection when a paddle device is unavailable. Adapted from reference (39).

2. Method (Fig. 17)
   a. Stick 0.5 cm of an 8- to 9-cm-long strip of tape to one end of a slide. Run the remaining tape around the end and onto the top of the slide with the gummed side down so that the tape extends beyond the other end of the slide for about 1 cm. Fold the extended end in half so that the two gummed sides stick to each other and form a tab that is not stuck to the slide.

b. Hold the slide against the tongue depressor, grasp the tab at the end of the tape, and lift the long part of the tape up from the slide.

c. Loop the tape over the end of the depressor so that the gummed surface of the tape is exposed.

d. Hold the tape and the slide against the depressor to provide firm support for the tape.

e. Separate the patient's buttocks and press the gummed surface against several areas of the perianal region.

f. Restick the tape onto the slide.

g. Smooth the tape with cotton or gauze.

C. Labeling
1. Label the specimen with patient information.
2. Indicate the time of collection and the age of the patient.
3. Refrigerate the specimen.

D. Transport
1. Transport the specimen to the laboratory as quickly as possible.
2. Refrigerate the specimen after collection.

E. Comments
1. The larvae in *Enterobius* eggs deteriorate rapidly if exposed to heat.
2. To increase the chance of picking up eggs, use the tape procedure between 10 p.m. and midnight. Otherwise, early-morning testing is critical.
3. The collection of multiple specimens may be necessary.
4. Because the eggs are very infectious, observe aseptic technique and do not touch the sticky side of the tape after collecting the specimen.
5. Pediatric needs: This is usually a pediatric specimen and is collected as described above.

## Rectal and Anal Swab Specimens

A. Selection (In most cases, the specimen of choice for culture of a bacterial agent of diarrhea is a portion of a diarrheal stool, not material on a swab.)
   1. Rectal swabs are acceptable only for culture of diarrheal pathogens from infants or from patients who are acutely ill with diarrhea.
   2. Swabs for culture of enteric pathogens must show feces. Anal swabs are usually not acceptable for culture of bacterial agents of diarrhea.
   3. Routine culture usually indicates a search for *Salmonella*, *Shigella*, Shiga toxin-producing *E. coli*, and *Campylobacter* spp. If other agents are suspected, consult the laboratory.
   4. For group B streptococcus isolation, see "General Information" under "Genital Specimens" later in this section.

B. Collection
   1. Materials
      a. Swab
      b. Transport medium
   2. Method
      a. Gently insert the swab beyond the anal sphincter, rotate it, remove it, and place it in transport medium. The swab should show feces.
      b. For *Neisseria gonorrhoeae* (GC) cultures, swab the anal crypts just inside the anal ring. Avoid fecal contamination as much as possible.
      c. Place the GC swab in transport medium immediately or inoculate a special GC plate at the patient's bedside or at the examination table. Consult the laboratory about the appropriate medium to use.

C. Labeling
   1. Label the sample with patient information.
   2. Indicate the pathogens sought, especially if GC is suspected.
   3. Indicate the time of collection on the requisition form.

D. Transport
   1. For *N. gonorrhoeae*, do not refrigerate the specimen, but deliver it to the laboratory within 30 min of collection if possible.
   2. For routine culture, refrigerate the transport medium if a delay in transit of 6 h or more is anticipated.

**E.** Comments
   1. The specimen of choice for diagnosing the bacterial agent of diarrhea is the diarrheal stool, not a formed stool. An acceptable stool sample is one that takes the shape of the container.
   2. *Neisseria gonorrhoeae* is fastidious and dies at refrigerator temperatures, without carbon dioxide, or without its proper culture medium.
   3. If organisms such as *Yersinia* spp., and in some cases, *Vibrio* spp. and *Aeromonas* or *Plesiomonas* spp. are suspected, notify the laboratory.
   4. A rectal swab is not recommended for detection of the toxin of *Clostridium difficile*. In addition, formed stools should not be accepted for testing.
   5. Pediatric needs: Collection and transport are essentially the same as for adults. Consider the need in the local area for culture of *Yersinia enterocolitica* and *Aeromonas hydrophila*. Swabs for use with antigen detection enzyme-linked immunosorbent assays are acceptable as long as feces are visible on the swab.

## Sigmoidoscopy Specimens for Amebiasis

**A.** Selection
   1. Sigmoidoscopy is used when amebiasis is suspected but stool specimens have been negative for parasite studies.
   2. Do not use catharsis, an enema, or barium before a sigmoidoscopy. If catharsis is necessary, wait 2 to 3 h before doing the procedure.
   3. Take material directly from the intestinal mucosa, where amebas are likely to be attached or embedded.

**B.** Collection
   1. Materials
      a. Serologic pipette with rubber bulb
      b. Curette (if scraping is to be done)
      c. Endoscope or sigmoidoscope
   2. Method
      a. Gently insert the lubricated sigmoidoscope into the rectum.
      b. Pass the instrument to the point where the sigmoid colon can be seen.
      c. With a serologic pipette, aspirate material from visible lesions and from the mucosal surface.
      d. A curette can be used to gently scrape suspicious areas of the mucosal wall. Cotton-tipped swabs are *not* recommended because they absorb too much material.
      e. Place the sample in a sterile culture tube and deliver it to the laboratory immediately.

**C.** Labeling
   1. Label the specimen with patient information.
   2. Indicate the exact specimen source, e.g., "lesion from sigmoid colon" or "sigmoidoscopy."
   3. Indicate whether occult blood or other studies are needed.

**D.** Transport
   1. Rapid transport is essential.
   2. Do *not* refrigerate the specimen.

**E.** Comments
   1. Unless something else is requested, only an examination for amebiasis should be done.
   2. Collect as much material as possible and prevent it from drying. Rapid transport of the specimen to the laboratory increases the success of observation.
   3. Three stool specimens may still be needed to confirm a diagnosis.
   4. Pediatric needs: Same as for adults.

## ◼ Stool or Feces for Culture or Parasitology Studies

**A.** Selection
   1. The specimen of choice is a diarrheal stool (the acute stage of illness).
   2. A rectal swab for bacterial culture *must* show feces. In general, swabs are recommended only for infants.
   3. For bacterial pathogens, collect and submit three specimens, one each day for 3 days. For parasite examination by microscopy, three specimens collected every other day or every third day should be adequate. A single stool specimen may not exclude bacterial or parasitic pathogens as a cause of diarrhea except when an enzyme immunoassay is used to detect *Giardia* antigen.
   4. To rule out the carrier state for some organisms, three consecutive *negative* specimens are often needed.
   5. Specimens for parasite examination collected too soon after the administration of barium, oil, magnesium, or crystalline compounds are unsatisfactory. Delay specimen collection for a minimum of 5 days after administration of these agents.

**B.** Collection
   1. Materials
      a. Commode collection systems in which a plastic collection device fits over the rim of a toilet seat are available (Fig. 18). Alternatively, a clean, waxed cardboard cup with a secure lid or some other similar container (when the specimen is for bacterial culture and immediate parasite examination) can be used. The smaller the container, the more difficult it is for the patient to provide an appropriate specimen.
      b. Swab (for acutely ill patients or when a stool specimen is not available)
      c. Parasitology transport pack (one jar of formalin, one jar of polyvinyl alcohol) or the equivalent (Fig. 19).
   2. Method
      a. Instruct patients who can to excrete directly into the cup or collection device. Never take a specimen from the water in a toilet and do not allow urine to contaminate the specimen. Replace the lid tightly and refrigerate the specimen.
      b. Alternatively, collect feces from a sterile bedpan, plastic wrap, or paper, and place 10 to 20 g in the container.
      c. For parasite studies, use either method described above and then transport the specimen *directly* to the laboratory while it is still warm. If a delay is necessary, place about 0.5 to 1 teaspoon of specimen in each fixative provided (Fig. 20).

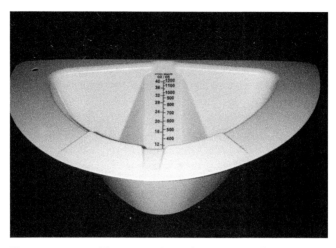

**Figure 18** Disposable sanitary device for collection of stool speci-mens. Oral and written directions for specimen timing, preservation, and transport to the laboratory should be provided to the patient.

C. Labeling
   1. Label the specimen with patient information.
   2. Indicate the type of studies required: routine culture, ovum and parasite, special studies, etc.
   3. Indicate the time and date of collection.
   4. Indicate any special patient history (travel, other ill family members, etc.).
   5. Label as a specimen in a series for a single patient if appropriate (e.g., "1 of 3," "2 of 3," "3 of 3").

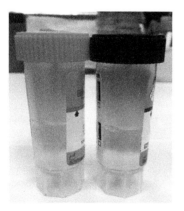

**Figure 19**  For parasitology studies, patients must be given one or two special transport vials and directions for their use.

*Note:* Both soft and formed specimens should be submitted by this method. Specimens must be *fresh* when placed in vials.

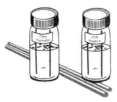

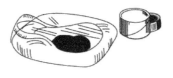

**1** The kit consists of two vials (one with 10% formalin and one with PVA fixative).

**2** The stool should be passed into a dry container. Urine should not be passed into the same container.

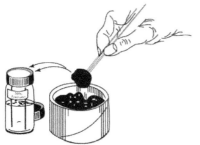

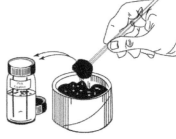

**3** Using applicator sticks, place a quantity of the stool into the 10% formalin (ratio of 3 parts formalin to 1 part stool).

**4** Place a similar quantity into the vial containing the PVA fixative.

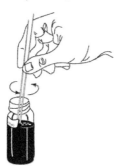

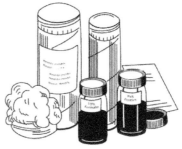

**5** Thoroughly break up specimen in the 10% formalin and PVA fixative. Shake vigorously.

**6** Pack the two vials so as to protect against breakage. Enclose appropriate identification and mail or deliver to laboratory.

**Figure 20** Illustrated instructions on how to use the parasitology transport and preservative vial(s) may be helpful to patients. A non-mercury-containing fixative may be used in place of polyvinyl alcohol (PVA). Adapted from reference 39.

**D.** Transport
1. If the specimen is not transported immediately for bacterial culture, refrigerate it.
2. If the specimen is to be submitted for *C. difficile* study and a >48-h delay is anticipated, freeze the specimen or submit it quickly at 4°C.
3. Submit fresh specimens for parasite studies as quickly as possible. Preserved specimens need not be rushed to the laboratory.
4. For bacterial pathogens, add the specimen to Cary-Blair transport medium if a 2- to 3-h delay is anticipated.

**E.** Comments
1. The laboratory must be notified if bacteria other than *Salmonella*, Shigella, Shiga toxin-producing *E. coli*, or *Campylobacter* spp. are suspected as the cause of diarrhea. Isolation of *Vibrio*, *Yersinia*, or *Aeromonas* spp. requires special laboratory procedures and is usually more expensive.
2. Susceptibility studies are not routinely done on isolates of *Campylobacter* spp.
3. Anaerobic studies are *not* done on feces.
4. Transport bile, colostomy, and ileostomy specimens in the same manner as other fecal specimens.
5. Small-bowel aspirates can be tested for anaerobes. *Bacteroides* and *Bifidobacterium* spp. can colonize the small bowel and cause a malabsorption syndrome in the presence of an obstruction.
6. Many laboratories offer an initial rapid parasite screening for *G. lamblia*, and perhaps *Cryptosporidium* spp., rather than a complete ovum and parasite microscopic examination. Modern enzyme immunoassay detection methods make it unnecessary, in most cases, to provide three fecal samples. Many studies have shown that one sample is usually enough to detect antigens.
7. The more immunosuppressed a patient is, the more likely it is that some parasites may disseminate to other body sites, requiring additional clinical specimens to be sent to the laboratory.
8. Pediatric needs: Essentially the same as for adults. Since children cannot reliably collect specimens in transport containers, the use of devices that fit into the toilet bowl or of procedures such as lining a diaper with plastic wrap facilitates retrieval of feces for testing. If the stool volume is small, adjust the parasite transport solution to retain the recommended stool to fixative ratio of 3:1. Rectal swabs are not recommended for ova and parasite examination.

## ▨ Stool Specimen Collection Directions
(Example to give to a patient or to read over the telephone)

The doctor has asked that you provide the laboratory with a stool specimen to determine what can be causing your problem. It is important that you follow these instructions carefully when collecting the specimen and bringing it to the laboratory.

1.  Try to deliver the specimen to the laboratory or doctor's office within 2 hours of the time you pass it. If possible, collect the specimen just before you come to the laboratory.

2.  The laboratory must have an amount of stool about the size of a small chicken egg.

3.  When you go to the bathroom, take with you what you will need to collect the specimen.
    a.  The doctor may have given you one or more special containers. If not, you can use a dry, clean, screw-cap jar such as a baby food jar or a clean, empty pint jar of some kind or even a clean plastic margarine container with a lid.
    b.  You will also need newspaper or plastic wrap and a tablespoon (a plastic utensil is fine) or a clean stick.

4.  Do not pass the specimen into the toilet and then dip it out. Either pass it directly into the container *or* pass it onto the newspaper *or* plastic wrap and then spoon an egg-size portion into the container. You can place the plastic wrap across the toilet under the lid or put the newspaper on the floor.

5.  If you were given one or two small containers with liquid in them labeled "formalin" or "PVA," place in each container an amount of stool about the size of a large marble and mix it *vigorously* with a stick or a spoon handle. *These liquids are poisonous. Do not drink them and do not let children play with them. Remember, mix well and replace the cap correctly and tightly.*

6. The sooner you can deliver the specimen to the laboratory, the better. If you cannot get there within 2 hours of the time you obtained the specimen, place the sealed container in your refrigerator until you can get to the laboratory. The laboratory cannot use a specimen that was collected the day before.

7. If the doctor asked you to provide three specimens, wait 48 hours between stool collections (28). *Be sure to label the container with the date the specimen was collected.*

# GENITAL SPECIMENS

## General Information

**A.** Because genital specimens are often taken from sites harboring large numbers of commensal (normal) flora, attention to specimen selection and collection methods is critical.

**B.** Routine vaginal specimens for culture are discouraged because the presence of high numbers of commensal flora makes them difficult to interpret. Diagnosis of vaginosis/vaginitis can often made by Gram stain, not culture (30).

**C.** Anaerobic studies are limited to certain specimens, as shown in Table 13.

**D.** Many agents of genital infection in women are limited to specific sites, some of which are listed in Table 14.

**E.** In the United States, *Chlamydia trachomatis* infections are more common than those caused by *N. gonorrhoeae*. The laboratory can detect *C. trachomatis* by direct microscopic examination, enzyme immunoassays, special culture, or the use of DNA probes. It is recommended that chlamydia tests be ordered with each GC request since the two infections often occur together and the symptoms mimic each other.

**F.** Bartholin's gland. Pus from gland abscesses can sometimes be collected from the Bartholin's ducts with digital palpation. Otherwise, material can be aspirated directly by needle and syringe.

**Table 13** Genital specimens for culture

| Source | Specimen or source | |
|---|---|---|
| | Not cultured for anaerobes | Cultured for anaerobes |
| Females | Endocervix | Placenta from cesarean section |
| | Vagina | Uterus (endometrium) |
| | Urethra | Fallopian tube |
| | Placenta | Cervical aspirate |
| | Vulva | Ovary |
| | Female genital | Bartholin's gland |
| | Lochia | |
| | Perineum | |
| Males | Urethra | |
| | Prostatic fluid | |
| | Seminal fluid | |

**Table 14**  Agents of genital infection in women

| Site of infection | Organism possibly involved |
| --- | --- |
| Vulva | *Treponema pallidum*<br>*Haemophilus ducreyi*<br>*Chlamydia* spp.<br>Herpesvirus<br>Yeasts |
| Vagina | *Trichomonas vaginalis*<br>*Candida albicans*<br>Mixed bacteria of bacterial vaginosis |
| Cervix | *N. gonorrhoeae*<br>*Chlamydia* spp.<br>Herpesvirus<br>*Actinomyces* spp. |
| Urethra, upper tract | *N. gonorrhoeae*<br>*Chlamydia* spp.<br>Aerobic and anaerobic bacteria |

**G.** Endometrium. Specimens are best obtained by suction curette. They should not be collected through the cervix with an unprotected swab because they will be contaminated by cervical and vaginal flora, the same bacteria that cause endometritis.

**H.** Pelvic inflammatory disease. All specimens are obtained by invasive techniques. Peritoneal fluid can be collected from the cul-de-sac by aspiration through the posterior vaginal vault (culdocentesis). Material taken directly from the fallopian tubes or ovaries is collected surgically.

**I.** Scrapings, aspirates, and biopsy material from vulvar lesions are usually of no value except in cases of syphilis. When there are syphilitic lesions, collect specimens by carefully abrading the lesion with dry gauze until serous fluid is expressed (avoid causing bleeding because it interferes with dark-field microscopic interpretation). After the fluid has accumulated, place one drop on a clean slide and examine it immediately for motile spirochetes.

**J.** Intrauterine devices. These devices are removed surgically to prevent cervical or vaginal contamination. Place the entire device, including any exudate, in a sterile container for transport to the laboratory.

K. Chlamydial infections. Do *not* submit vaginal secretions because the organism cannot grow in the squamous epithelial cells lining the vagina; thus, it does not cause vaginitis. *Chlamydiae* are obligate intracellular parasites of the columnar cells of the cervix. Collect these cells by briskly swabbing the endocervical area to obtain cells and secretions. Inoculate the swab immediately into special chlamydia transport medium or prepare a slide set for staining.

L. For detection of group B streptococci in women, new public health guidelines suggest obtaining one or two swabs of the vaginal introitus and the anorectum. Cervical cultures are not acceptable, and a speculum should not be used. Swabs can be placed safely in bacterial transport medium. The use of a selective broth or culture is recommended.

M. Prostatic secretions can be collected either by digital massage through the rectum and accompanied by pre- and postmassage urine specimens using the Meares and Stamey four-glass procedure (31) or the Nickel 2-glass procedure (32), or the ejaculate can be submitted for culture.

N. Pediatric needs: Calcium alginate swabs are appropriate for the collection of genital specimens in children. Genital specimens are usually obtained either for investigation of possible abuse or for diagnosis of premenarchal vulvovaginitis or urethritis. Since these specimens are often irretrievable, every effort must be made to process pediatric urogenital specimens for culture. Most sexually transmitted diseases in prepubertal girls involve the vagina rather than the cervix.

---

*Note:* For children who may be victims of sexual abuse, make sure a chain-of-possession form is available to document that the specimen received in the laboratory actually was collected from the patient named on the form.

## ▪ Cervical or Endocervical Specimens

**A.** Selection
1. Contamination of cervical or endocervical specimens with vaginal secretions interferes with the recovery of *N. gonorrhoeae* and invalidates interpretation by Gram staining.
2. Select only material from the endocervix by using a speculum to aid in examining the area.

**B.** Collection
1. Material
   a. Cervical speculum
   b. Swabs
   c. Transport medium
   d. Warm water
2. Method
   a. Moisten the speculum with warm water. Lubricants can be toxic to *Neisseria*.
   b. Look at the cervix and remove from the cervical os any mucous or vaginal material.
   c. Gently compress the cervix with the blades of the speculum and collect the endocervical discharge with a calcium alginate, Dacron, or nontoxic cotton swab or a flocked swab. Alternatively, insert the swab into the cervical os, allow it to remain in place for a few seconds, and remove it.
   d. Anal cultures can be collected to accompany cervical specimens when *N. gonorrhoeae* is suspected. The rectum may be the only positive post-treatment site. Insert a swab about 2.5 cm into the anal canal, just inside the anal ring. Move the swab from side to side and then remove it. *No fecal material should be on the swab.*

**C.** Labeling
1. Label the specimen with patient information.
2. Indicate the suspected diagnosis.
3. Indicate the time the specimen was collected and its specific source.

**D.** Transport
1. Although *N. gonorrhoeae* can survive on swabs for up to 6 h, viability is inevitably lost over time.
2. Specimens to be cultured for GC must be cultured immediately and placed in $CO_2$.

3. Ideally, the swab specimen is inoculated directly onto special media at the patient's bedside. Otherwise, place the swab in transport medium and deliver it to the laboratory promptly.

4. Do *not* refrigerate the specimen.

E. Comment

1. Gram staining cannot be used effectively to detect *N. gonorrhoeae* in vaginal or cervical specimens. Other commensal organisms that morphologically mimic this agent are present.

2. Pediatric needs: Same as for adults; however, collection from the cervix for culture is appropriate only in adolescent (pubescent) populations.

> *If cervical mucus is not thoroughly removed prior to endocervical specimen collection, neither a cytobrush nor a scraper used to collect the specimen, nor an amplification assay to detect the pathogen, will result in adequate detection of* Chlamydia trachomatis *or an accurate determination of its prevalence.*
>
> JIM KELLOGG, Ph.D.
> York Hospital, York, PA

## ■ Genital Smears for Herpes

**A.** Selection
1. Select vesicle fluid and the bases of lesions for collection.
2. Endocervical and vaginal wall specimens are acceptable.

**B.** Collection
1. Materials
   a. Virus transport system
   b. Swab (calcium alginate may not be suitable)
   c. Tuberculin syringe with a 26-gauge needle
   d. Scalpel blade (for removing lesion surface)
2. Method (for three sites)
   a. Vesicles: Visually locate the vesicle and aseptically aspirate its contents with the needle and syringe. Sample the base of a lesion with a swab.
   b. Cervix: Insert a swab into the endocervix and rotate it gently.
   c. Vagina: Swab the vaginal walls.

**C.** Labeling
1. Label the specimen with patient information and the *exact* specimen source.
2. Indicate that herpesvirus is being sought and if medical history includes herpesvirus infection.
3. Indicate the time of collection.

**D.** Transport
1. Refrigerate but *do not freeze the specimen.*
2. Transport the specimen to the laboratory with the swab inserted in a viral transport vial or container. Do *not* use bacterial transport medium.

**E.** Comments
1. Prevent bacterial contamination as much as possible. Hold the specimen at refrigerator temperature. Do not freeze it or hold it at room temperature. The container can be immersed in wet ice.
2. Freezing and subsequent thawing of any specimen submitted for viral culture may destroy virions, thus preventing successful culture in the laboratory.
3. Pediatric needs: Same as for adults.

## Urethral and Penile Specimens

**A.** Selection
1. The urethra is the male genital site most commonly cultured.
2. Remove the external skin flora of the urethral meatus as in preparation for obtaining a urine specimen.
3. Material from a site about 2 cm inside the urethra (collected by swab) or expressed pus is the specimen of choice.
4. Many facilities and offices now use nucleic acid amplification tests to detect *N. gonorrhoeae* and thus require only a urine specimen, not a urethral swab.

**B.** Collection for urethral swab
1. Materials
   a. Urethrogenital swab
   b. Transport medium
   c. Slide for stained smear
2. Method
   a. Express exudate from the urethra and collect it on a swab. Place the swab in transport medium.
   b. Collect additional exudate on a swab and use this swab to prepare a slide for staining. Roll the swab over 2 to 3 cm of the slide surface and label the same side.
   c. If exudate is unavailable, insert a urethrogenital swab about 2 cm into the urethra, gently rotate it, and remove it.
   d. Inoculate the specimen onto special medium as soon as possible and place the specimen in a $CO_2$ atmosphere at 35°C. After plating, prepare a smear for staining. If two swabs are available, submit one for culture and prepare a smear with the other.

**C.** Labeling
1. Label the specimen with patient information.
2. Indicate the time of collection.
3. Indicate the suspected diagnosis.

**D.** Transport
1. Do *not* refrigerate the specimen.
2. Transport the specimen to the laboratory immediately.

E. Comments
1. Diagnosis of gonorrhea in males can often be confirmed by Gram staining of urethral exudate. For females, confirmation by Gram staining of GC in vaginal or cervical secretions is not possible because some nonpathogenic species in the vagina may resemble the diplococcal morphology of *N. gonorrhoeae.*
2. *Neisseria gonorrhoeae* is nutritionally fastidious and environmentally fragile and cannot tolerate cold temperatures or the lack of $CO_2$.
3. Along with the test for *N. gonorrhoeae,* consider a request for chlamydia detection because this agent is often found in patients with urethritis.
4. The choice of swab type is critical. Check the package insert or contact the laboratory to determine whether cotton-, calcium alginate-, or Dacron-tipped or flocked swabs should be used with the selected procedure.
5. Pediatric needs: Same as for adults.

# RESPIRATORY SPECIMENS

## General Information

A. Upper respiratory tract infections
1. These infections are subdivided into pharyngitis, laryngitis, epiglottitis, and sinusitis.
2. Each infection is characteristically caused by certain organisms that dictate specific requirements for the collection and transport of specimens.
3. Pharyngitis
   a. Acute cases may yield beta-hemolytic streptococci by culture or group A streptococci only by direct antigen detection. It is important to understand the limits of detection of direct antigen tests.
   b. Culture for *N. gonorrhoeae* in the throat is not a routine request. Indicate this special request on the requisition and plate the specimen immediately if possible. This organism dies rapidly at refrigerator temperature. Gram staining cannot be used to identify it from throat specimens.
   c. Collect specimens for *Corynebacterium diphtheriae* testing by swabbing the posterior nares. Also sample the posterior pharynx. Use a routine transport medium.
   d. For viral agents, sample the throat with a swab or obtain nasal washings. Submit the specimen in viral transport medium.
4. Laryngitis
   a. This infection is primarily caused by viruses such as parainfluenza virus, respiratory syncytial virus, influenza virus, and adenovirus.
   b. If necessary for diagnosis, sample the throat with a swab or obtain nasal washings. Submit the specimen in viral transport medium.
5. Epiglottitis
   a. Culture of the throat is *not* indicated. Touching the inflamed epiglottis may precipitate complete obstruction of the airway.
   b. The specimen of choice, if one is necessary, is blood for culture.
6. Sinusitis
   a. The specimen of choice is a needle aspirate from the sinuses obtained after decontamination of the nasal cavity. Do not submit a swab.
   b. No specimen other than an aspirate is recommended.

B. Lower respiratory tract infections
1. Careful specimen collection is important because there is always a degree of contamination of the specimen with oropharyngeal flora, thus making the results clinically irrelevant.

2. Multiple tests cannot be performed on small-volume specimens such as aspirates or biopsy samples.
3. Specimen quality is judged microscopically (Fig. 21). A properly collected specimen containing a minimum of squamous epithelial cells and significant numbers of polymorphonuclear leukocytes usually provides clinically relevant results. Specimens of lesser quality provide misleading results and should not be interpreted. Allow the microbiology laboratory to offer input.
4. *Bordetella pertussis* is a fastidious organism requiring immediate culture. The specimen of choice is mucus from the posterior nasopharynx. A special transport medium such as Regan-Lowe or Jones-Kendrick medium must be ordered and used. Respiratory therapy personnel may assist in obtaining nasopharyngeal washings.

**Figure 21** Specimen quality is judged microscopically. The presence of epithelial cells usually signals the presence of commensal flora that can confuse accurate interpretation.

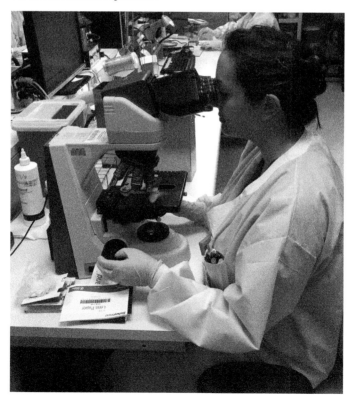

## Bronchoscopy-Bronchial Washing

**A.** Selection
1. Collect the specimen via a bronchoscope.
2. Directly sample the lower respiratory tract.
3. The involved area of the lung must be accessible.
4. Bronchial brushings are preferable to washings because washings are more dilute.

**B.** Collection
1. Materials
   a. Lidocaine (2%) (preferred) for anesthesia
   b. Lactated Ringer's solution or saline for bronchial brush specimens
   c. A double-lumen bronchoscope with a telescoping double catheter with a distal polyethylene glycol plug can be used.
   d. Lukens trap for containing the specimen (Fig. 22)
   e. 20-ml Luer slip syringe
   f. Disposable cytology brush
   g. Xylocaine (4%)

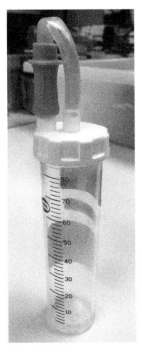

**Figure 22** A Lukens trap is used for collecting many respiratory aspirates.

2. Method
   a. Anesthetize the area by having the patient inhale via a mouthpiece and exhale through the nose. Lubricate both nares with xylocaine jelly. The patient may also need an intravenous sedative to tolerate the bronchoscopy.
   b. Tilt the patient back into a semi-Fowler's position.
   c. Lubricate the bronchoscope with 2% xylocaine jelly, avoiding the distal tip.
   d. Introduce the bronchoscope transnasally.
   e. For bronchial washings (a poor predictor of agents of pneumonia)
      i. Attach the Lukens trap to the bronchoscope.
      ii. Instill 10 ml of nonbacteriostatic saline through the channel opening.
      iii. Suction material out.
      iv. Seal the Lukens tube and submit it to the laboratory.
   f. For bronchial brushings, double lumen
      i. Insert the cytology brush unit into the channel opening of the scope and advance it.
      ii. Push the brush out of its sheath and obtain brushings.
      iii. Pull the brush back into the sheath and withdraw the entire brush unit. Brushings air-dry rapidly, and this drying is detrimental to successful culture.
      iv. Snip the brush from the unit, placing it in transport liquid such as saline or Ringer's lactate. For mycobacterial specimens, place the material in 10 ml of Middlebrook 7H9 broth supplemented with 1 to 2% (final concentration) bovine serum albumin and 0.5% Tween 80.
      v. Submit the specimen to the laboratory.
      vi. Pediatric needs: Same as for adults.
   g. For bronchoalveolar lavage (specimen of choice)
      i. Lavage is used to wash cells out of small airways that bronchoscopy cannot reach.
      ii. Attach a 70-ml specimen trap to the bronchoscope.
      iii. Forcefully instill 100 ml of nonbacteriostatic saline through the channel in 20-ml increments.

      In pediatric patients, only 1 to 2 ml/kg can be instilled. Usually, less than 10 ml is recovered in children. If more than 10 ml is collected, centrifugation of the sample improves the success of both culture and staining.
      iv. After the third or fourth instillation, replace the 70-ml trap with a 40-ml trap.

     v.  Submit the traps (labeled 1 [70 ml] or 2 [40 ml]) or aseptically remove 10 ml of fluid from each trap, place the fluid in sterile tubes, and submit the specimens to the laboratory.
- h. For a transbronchial lung biopsy (acid-fast bacillus and fungal culture)
  - i. Perform the procedure in the X-ray department under fluoroscopy.
  - ii. Slowly advance the biopsy forceps to the end of the channel.
  - iii. Move the forceps out of the channel and into the lung area.
  - iv. Initiate fluoroscopy.
  - v. Move the forceps to within 2.5 cm of the pleura. Open the forceps and push them into the lung. Close the forceps to obtain a specimen. Generally, three biopsy specimens are needed.
  - vi. Remove the forceps from the channel, keeping them closed.
  - vii. Place the tissue in a tube of saline (1 to 2 ml) and send it to the laboratory for acid-fast bacillus or fungal culture.

**C.** Labeling
1. Label the specimen trap or tube with patient information.
2. Include the procedure performed and the time of collection.
3. Specify the type of culture required: routine, acid-fast bacillus, or fungal.

**D.** Transport
1. Do *not* refrigerate the specimen.
2. Transport the specimen to the laboratory quickly.

**E.** Comments
1. Inhibition of bacteria by the anesthetic solution can be a major problem with bronchial washings because 90% or more of the collected material may contain anesthetic, rendering the specimen worthless.
2. Only about 0.001 ml of specimen is obtained with bronchial brushings. Unless this material is immediately transferred to a transport fluid, rapid loss of bacteria will result from desiccation of the specimen.
3. The specimen collection procedure must be guided with great technical skill.
4. Specimens collected via bronchoscopy are contaminated with oral microbial flora. The numbers of this flora can be greatly reduced by collecting secretions with a triple-lumen bronchoscope.
5. Most bronchoscopy specimens are *not* cultured for anaerobes. Consult the laboratory if special tests are to be requested.
6. Bronchoalveolar lavage specimens may be preferred after an initial sputum culture is unsuccessful. Quantitative analysis of lavage specimens is clinically more relevant than analysis of sputum specimens.

## Nasal Specimens

A. Selection
  1. The specimen of choice is a swab specimen taken at least 1 cm inside the nares.
  2. Lesions in the nose require samples from the advancing margin of the lesion.

B. Collection
  1. Materials
     a. Swab and transport medium set
     b. Nasal speculum (for some patients)
  2. Method
     a. Carefully insert the swab at least 1 cm into the nares.
     b. Firmly sample the membrane by rotating the swab and leaving it in place for 10 to 15 s.
     c. Withdraw the swab, insert it in a transport container, and crush the vial of transport medium in the container.

C. Labeling
  1. Label the swab container with patient information.
  2. Indicate whether a lesion is present.

D. Transport
  1. Transport the specimen to the laboratory as soon as possible.
  2. Do *not* refrigerate the specimen.

E. Comments
  1. Anterior nares cultures, without an indication of the presence of a lesion, are routinely examined *only* for *Staphylococcus aureus* and beta-hemolytic streptococci.
  2. Nasal cultures do *not* predict the etiologic agent of a sinus, middle ear, or lower respiratory tract infection and should not be submitted in lieu of specimens from these sites.
  3. Anaerobic cultures are not done on nasal specimens.
  4. Detection of carriage of MRSA can be increased by also sampling another body site, such as the rectum. Two or three consecutively negative samples from these areas usually indicate that the patient is free from carriage. In any case, the presence of MRSA in a patient should not preclude the patient's admission or readmission to a nursing home or hospital.

5. Pediatric needs: For nasal washing, place about 4 ml of sterile saline in a 1-oz tapered rubber bulb. Tilt the patient's head back about 70°, insert the bulb into the nose until the nostril is occluded, and squeeze the bulb to dispense the saline. Hold for a few seconds and then release the bulb to reaspirate the fluid. Transfer the fluid to a sterile container and transport it to the laboratory immediately. Specimens for viral culture should be transported on ice.

## ▦ Nasopharyngeal Specimens

A. Selection
1. Specimens must be taken in a way that avoids contamination with nasal or oral flora.
2. The nasopharynx can be reached by inserting a small nasopharyngeal swab through either the nose or the throat.

B. Collection
1. Materials
   a. Nasal speculum (optional)
   b. Nasopharyngeal swab with transport medium
   c. A special transport medium such as Regan-Lowe medium is necessary if whooping cough is suspected. Alert the laboratory early.
2. Method
   a. Remove excess secretions or exudate from the anterior nares.
   b. Insert the nasal speculum if one is to be used.
   c. Gently pass the swab through the nose and into the nasopharynx, a distance about halfway between the ear and the base of the nose (Fig. 23).

**Figure 23**  Nasopharyngeal specimens are often collected inadequately. To reach the nasopharynx, the swab should be inserted approximately half the distance from the base of the nose to the ear.

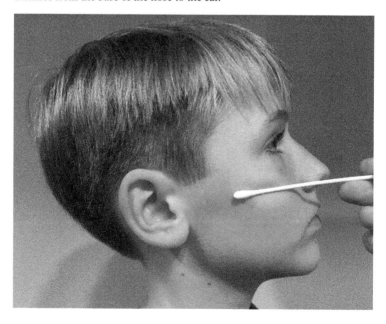

d. Rotate the swab on the nasopharyngeal membrane and allow it to remain in place for 10 to 15 s to absorb organisms.

e. Remove the swab carefully and place it in the transport medium. Do *not* refrigerate it.

f. Remove the speculum.

g. Alternatively, bend the wire at an angle and insert it into the throat. Then move the swab upward into the nasopharyngeal space.

C. Labeling
1. Label the specimen with patient information.
2. Include the suspected diagnosis where possible, especially if whooping cough (pertussis) is suspected.

D. Transport
1. Do *not* refrigerate the specimen.
2. Transport the specimen to the laboratory quickly.

E. Comments
1. Nasopharyngeal specimens should *not* be used to detect the agent causing a sinus infection (Fig. 24).

**Figure 24**  Diagram of the nose and nasopharyngeal region. While nasal and nasopharyngeal specimens may be obtained by swab, a needle aspirate is the specimen of choice for determining the etiologic agent(s) of sinusitis.

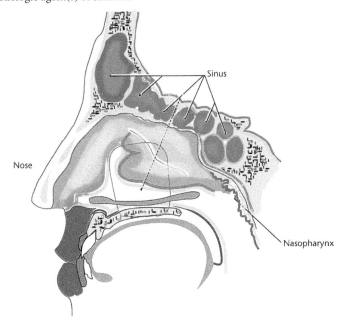

2. Nasopharyngeal specimens are cultured primarily to detect meningo-coccal carriers or to diagnose whooping cough.
3. The use of the small-tipped nasopharyngeal swabs for routine bacterial culture is not recommended.
4. Specimens received on large-tipped (Culturette-type) swabs are assumed to be from the nose and not the nasopharynx, regardless of the source given on the specimen label.
5. Pediatric needs: For a nasopharyngeal aspirate, attach a sterile suction catheter to a Lukens trap and introduce the end of the catheter into the nasopharynx until resistance is encountered. Withdraw the catheter 1 to 2 cm and apply suction to aspirate a sample.

## ▨ Sputum

A. Selection
1. Sputum may *not* be the best specimen for determining the etiologic agent of bacterial pneumonia. Blood specimens, lavage specimens, or transtracheal aspirates may be more accurate.
2. Lower respiratory tract secretions from infected patients are confirmed by noting the presence of large numbers of leukocytes in the absence of epithelial cells. Since epithelial cells in the specimen signal gross contamination with oropharyngeal flora, culture only specimens that represent infection.
3. Careful attention to the instructions given the patient greatly reduces the number of inappropriate specimens.
4. The first early-morning specimen is preferred. Pooled specimens are not recommended for culture. Pooled specimens may only dilute the true etiologic agent.
5. Handle all lower respiratory tract specimens with the safety precautions necessary for working with *M. tuberculosis*.

B. Collection
1. Materials
   a. Sterile screw-cap sputum collection cup (Fig. 25)
2. Method
   a. Instruct the patient in the difference between sputum and spit. Explain that a deep cough the first thing in the morning, if practical, is needed to produce a sputum sample.
   b. Have the patient rinse the mouth with water. For patients with dentures, remove the dentures first. Have the patient take two to three deep breaths prior to coughing.
   c. Collect the specimen directly in the container. True sputum will be thick, not a thin liquid.
   d. Carefully and tightly replace the cap. Be careful not to misthread the lid because leakage will occur, thus signaling the laboratory to discard the entire container before culture. Check the cap to ensure that it is secure.
   e. Submit the capped tube containing the specimen and discard the outer package.

C. Labeling
1. Label the specimen with patient information.
2. Indicate whether the specimen is for routine, acid-fast bacillus, or fungal culture.

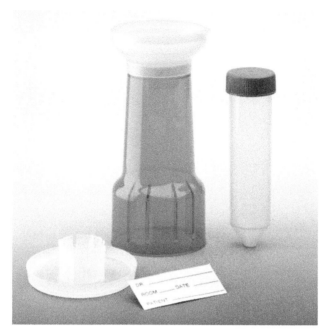

**Figure 25** Sterile, prepackaged sputum collection containers are provided to patients along with oral and written instructions on how to collect an appropriate specimen. In this system, sputum is collected in the funnel-shaped device. The tube that contains the specimen is removed, and the cap is firmly applied.

**D.** Transport
1. Refrigerate the specimen if a delay of more than 1 to 2 h is anticipated.
2. Transport the specimen to the laboratory quickly.

**E.** Comments
1. A single properly collected specimen should be adequate for the diagnosis of bacterial lower respiratory tract disease.
2. For the diagnosis of fungal or mycobacterial disease, separately process three consecutive early-morning specimens. Culture of more than five specimens a week for these agents is not indicated.
3. Anaerobic studies of sputum are not done.
4. Direct tests using DNA probes may be available. Check with the laboratory about other rapid or molecular tests that may be available.
5. Pediatric needs: Same as for adults. Since children are often unable to produce sputum, tracheal aspirates are more often collected in pediatric populations.

## Tracheal Aspirate

A. Selection
   1. The specimen of choice for diagnosing pneumonia should be blood for culture or a transtracheal aspirate.
   2. Process the specimen as sputum is processed.
   3. Collect the specimen through a tracheostomy or endotracheal tube.

B. Collection
   1. Materials
      a. Polyethylene catheter, to pass into the site
      b. Syringe (20 ml) or intermittent suction device
   2. Method
      a. Carefully pass the catheter through the site and into the trachea.
      b. Aspirate material from the trachea using the syringe or an intermittent suction device.
      c. Remove the catheter and disengage the syringe or device.

C. Labeling
   1. Label the specimen with patient information.
   2. Give the specific source of the specimen.
   3. Indicate the suspected diagnosis and whether the patient is taking antimicrobial agents.

D. Transport
   1. Do *not* refrigerate the specimen.
   2. Transport the specimen to the laboratory quickly.

E. Comments
   1. Aspirates obtained through endotracheal tubes present the same problem as nasopharyngeal aspirates; the catheter must pass through densely colonized areas, making culture interpretation difficult.
   2. Since tracheostomy sites rapidly become colonized with Gram-negative bacteria, the presence of these organisms in a culture may or may not indicate the etiology of pneumonia. Thus, no real significance can be ascribed either to the presence of large numbers of an organism or to the organism's association with an inflammatory response.
   3. Prevent excessive dilution of the specimen with saline.
   4. Pediatric needs: After oxygenation of the patient, attach a sterile suction catheter to a Lukens trap and introduce the catheter into the endotracheal tract until resistance is encountered. Withdraw the catheter 1 to 2 cm and apply suction to aspirate the sample.

## Transtracheal Aspirate

A. Selection
  1. Transtracheal aspiration is a surgical procedure performed by a physician.
  2. Use this procedure when culture results will influence therapy, when non-invasive procedures have been nonproductive, when the infection is life threatening, when anaerobic infection is suspected, or when the patient is comatose.

B. Collection
  1. Materials
     a. Intracatheter needle (14 gauge) and polyethylene catheter (16 gauge)
     b. Syringe (20 ml) or intermittent suction device
     c. Anesthetic
     d. Alcohol and iodine preparations
  2. Method
     a. Anesthetize the skin over the collection site and prepare the site.
     b. Insert the needle through the cricothyroid membrane.
     c. Pass the catheter through the needle and into the lower trachea. Remove the needle.
     d. Aspirate secretions with the syringe or the suction device. Obtain as much fluid as possible with one syringe.
     e. If secretions are scant, inject 2 to 4 ml of sterile saline to induce coughing, which usually produces an adequate specimen.

C. Labeling
  1. Label the specimen with the exact source and with patient information.
  2. Indicate whether the specimen is to be tested for anaerobes or unusual agents.
  3. Do *not* refrigerate the specimen.

D. Transport
  1. Submit either the syringe containing the aspirate or the aspiration device with the tubing attached.
  2. Do not allow air to enter the transport container. Some anaerobic organisms are killed by oxygen.
  3. Submit the specimen to the laboratory quickly; fastidious agents may be involved.

E. Comments
  1. In cases of uncontrolled coughing, the catheter might be misdirected into the oropharynx. In this case, false-positive results may occur.
  2. The trachea below the larynx is normally sterile except in patients with chronic pulmonary disease or an endotracheal or tracheostomy tube.
  3. Pediatric needs: Same as for adults.

## ▨ Throat Specimens

**A.** Selection. Success with culture or with direct antigen detection depends on *firmly and completely* sampling an area of the inflamed throat.
  1. Using a tongue depressor to hold the tongue down, look at the back of the throat and the tonsillar area for localized areas of inflammation and exudate.
  2. These areas are the most productive for producing cultures of the etiologic agents of acute pharyngitis.

**B.** Collection
  1. Materials
    a. Dacron or calcium alginate swab or flocked swab and transport medium
    b. Tongue depressor
  2. Method
    a. Carefully but firmly rub the swab over several areas of exudate or over the tonsils and posterior pharynx (Fig. 26).
    b. Do not touch the cheeks, teeth, or gums with the swab as you withdraw it from the mouth.
    c. Insert the swab back into its packet and crush the transport medium vial in the transport container.

**C.** Labeling
  1. Label the swab container with patient identification data, including the time of collection.
  2. Note any antimicrobial agents currently being taken by the patient.
  3. Note whether the specimen is for culture, for direct antigen detection, or for a streptococcus screening procedure.
  4. Indicate the suspected pathogen if it is other than streptococci, e.g., *N. gonorrhoeae.*

**D.** Transport
  1. Transport the swab to the laboratory as soon as possible.
  2. If transport is to be delayed beyond 1 h, refrigerate the swab.

**E.** Comments
  1. A streptococcus screen by culture tests for and reports only the presence or absence of beta-hemolytic streptococci, including group A. A throat culture, in addition to revealing group A streptococci, reveals other beta-hemolytic streptococci, *Haemophilus* spp., and significant numbers of other potential respiratory pathogens, including *Streptococcus pneumoniae, Pseudomonas aeruginosa, Staphylococcus aureus, Arcanobacterium,* and other suspected pathogens as agreed on by the users.
  2. Any beta-hemolytic streptococci are routinely identified and reported. They are the primary cause of acute bacterial pharyngitis and need not be tested for susceptibility to antimicrobial agents.

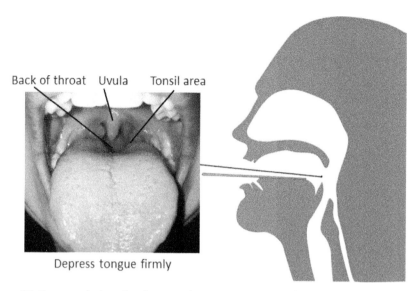

**Figure 26** Proper technique for obtaining throat specimens. Firmly sampling only the inflamed areas of the throat and tonsils and avoiding other oral sites will enhance detection of etiologic agents.

3. *Haemophilus* spp. can be reported in pediatric patients when requested, although they are part of the normal flora in children and adults.
4. Throat culture for *N. gonorrhoeae* is available on request, but the laboratory must be alerted to the request.
5. Routine susceptibility testing is not routinely done on any isolate from the throat, although a screen for MRSA may be requested if the carrier state for MRSA is suspected.
6. Pediatric needs: Same as for adults.

# URINE SPECIMENS

*Really, you squeezed that urine from the diaper and want us to culture it?*
Robert Jerris, Ph.D., (D)ABMM
Children's Healthcare of Atlanta, Atlanta, GA

## General Information

**A.** Our initial assumptions that urine is a sterile body fluid may or may not be true. In addition, urine may be transiently colonized with small numbers of organisms. Because urine is a good growth medium for many organisms, contamination of a urine specimen by organisms normally present in the urethra or on periurethral surfaces can allow a proliferation of these organisms that can cause misleading culture results.

**B.** For symptomatic patients (those with painful urination, urgency, or frequency), one specimen is usually adequate for diagnosis, and another is collected 48 to 72 h after institution of therapy. For asymptomatic patients, two or three specimens may be necessary. In cases of suspected renal tuberculosis, three consecutive first morning specimens should be submitted.

**C.** A pooled, 24-h collection of urine is unacceptable for culture, as is more than one specimen per 24 h.

**D.** The requisition form should indicate whether or not the patient is symptomatic. This information is critical to quantitative culture interpretation, especially of low-count urine specimens.

**E.** Urine held at room temperature supports the growth of both pathogens and contaminants. All urine *must* be refrigerated if it is not cultured within 30 min of collection. Refrigerated urine specimens should be cultured within 24 h.

**F.** Laboratories, in collaboration with the medical committee and specialists, may develop a reflex policy directing culture after a positive urinalysis. Such options must be clear on the requisition and physicians should be aware of these options.

## Urine from Catheters

A. Selection
   1. Urine collected by straight urethral catheterization is an acceptable specimen, but it can be associated with a small risk of causing bacteriuria because the urethral flora can be forced into the bladder during insertion of the catheter.
   2. Urine obtained from catheter bags at the bedside is unacceptable for culture.
   3. Material from Foley catheter tips is unacceptable for culture because these tips cannot be removed without picking up the urethral flora.
   4. Routine processing of urine from patients with chronic indwelling catheters may be of no value except epidemiologically. Large numbers of potential pathogens are common in such patients.
   5. The specimen of choice is urine collected from an indwelling catheter tube through the sampling port. Needleless urine sampling ports are now available to enhance safe practices when urine is collected from catheters.

B. Collection
   1. Materials
      a. 21-gauge needle and syringe
      b. Alcohol swabs
   2. Method
      a. If necessary, clamp the catheter tubing to collect urine in the tube but do not allow the clamp to remain for more than 30 min.
      b. Clean the sampling port (or tubing site if a port is unavailable) with alcohol swabs.
      c. Insert the needle into the tubing port and withdraw urine into the syringe.
      d. Transfer the urine to a sterile cup or tube.

C. Labeling
   1. Label the specimen with patient information.
   2. Indicate on the request form that the specimen was taken from an indwelling catheter.

D. Transport
   1. Refrigerate the urine if it will not be delivered to the laboratory within 30 min of collection.
   2. Place the specimen in the laboratory refrigerator if no one is in the laboratory to receive it.

**E.** Comments

1. Do not disconnect the catheter from the catheter bag to collect the specimen, and never submit bag contents for culture.
2. Patients with indwelling catheters are usually colonized after 48 to 72 h, often with multiple isolates. Biofilms play a significant role.
3. The laboratory must know whether the urine has been collected by any method that might introduce contamination: collection at home in an unconventional container or collection by an unknown method (e.g., from a nursing home).
4. Pediatric needs: Although suprapubic aspiration is the collection method of choice when retrieval of a specimen free of contamination is attempted, this method may not allow collection of the very small volumes of urine produced in the bladder by certain pediatric patients. For catheterization, a small-bore catheter is lubricated and gently inserted into the urethra until the bladder is reached and urine begins to flow. The first milliliter of urine, which may contain urethral contaminants, should be discarded. Even then, urethral contamination may be heavy in some specimens.

## Clean-Catch Urine

**A.** Selection

1. The first morning specimen is preferred.
2. Take the specimen *after* the first portion of urine has been voided. This first portion of the flow washes most contaminants from the urethra. The midstream portion represents the bladder flora.
3. In pediatric patients, initial screening is done by using a strapped-on bag device after careful cleaning as described below.

**B.** Collection

1. Materials

   a. Sterile screw-cap specimen container (Fig. 27A) and/or boric acid-containing tube for bacterial cultures (Fig. 27B)

   b. Antibacterial soap (ordinary soap is acceptable) or commercial preparatory packages. Some commercial antiseptic soaps and disinfectants may irritate the periurethral area and can inhibit bacterial growth on culture if they contaminate the collection cup.

   c. Gauze sponges

   d. Rinse water

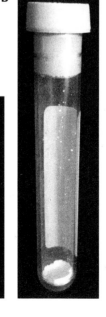

**Figure 27** Sterile, prepackaged urine collection cups are made available to patients, along with oral and written instructions (A). Urine can then be transferred to a special transport tube with preservatives (B); this step is usually performed by the health care personnel.

2. Method
   a. Supply the patient with clear oral and written instructions as follows. "We need a good urine specimen to diagnose your infection. It is important that you understand this procedure so that you will not contaminate the specimen with other germs."

   *Instructions for females*
   i.   Sit comfortably on the toilet and swing one knee to the side as far as you can.
   ii.  Spread yourself with one hand and hold yourself spread while you clean yourself and collect the specimen.
   iii. Wash. Be sure to wash and rinse well before you collect the specimen. Using the cleaning materials supplied, wipe your genital area as carefully as you can from the front to the back between the folds of skin.
   iv.  Rinse. After washing with each soap pad, rinse with a water-moistened pad with the same front-to-back motion. Use each pad only once and then throw it away.
   v.   Hold the cup with your fingers on the outside; do not touch the rim. First, pass a small amount of urine into the toilet and then pass enough urine into the cup to fill it half full.
   vi.  Place the lid on the cup carefully and tightly or ask the nurse to do it for you.

   *Instructions for males*
   i.   Retract the foreskin (if uncircumcised) and clean the glans (the head of the penis).
   ii.  Follow steps iii to vi above for cleaning yourself and collecting the urine.

   a. Check that the lid of the cup is secure and not misthreaded. A leaking container is dangerous to patients and personnel alike.
   b. Refrigerate the specimen if it will not be taken to the laboratory immediately (within 30 min).

C. Labeling
   1. Label the specimen with patient information.
   2. Indicate on the request form whether or not the patient is symptomatic and taking antibiotics.

D. Comments
   1. If a preservative tube will be used for bacterial culture orders, transfer the recommended amount of urine into the tube as soon after collection as possible. Store according to manufacturer's instructions until sent to the laboratory.

2. Culture urine from pediatric bags immediately to minimize interference by contaminants.
3. Routine urine samples are unacceptable for anaerobic culture.
4. Pediatric needs: With adult supervision, clean-catch urine specimens can be successfully collected from children as young as 3 years of age. As for adults, careful cleaning of the external urethra is essential. Although cleansing and midstream collection have been shown to have a questionable effect on the reduction of contaminants in the urine of children, such procedures enhance the quality of the specimen collected. For infants, a small sterile, plastic bag may be taped to the perineum after cleaning in order to retrieve a specimen during the next urination. Specimens obtained this way must be transported to the laboratory within 30 min of collection. Urine collected from disposable diapers cannot be reliably used for culture.

## Cystoscopic Specimens: Bilateral Urethral Catheterization

1. After adequate hydration, cystoscopy can begin.

2. Pass the cystoscope with its obturator in place into the bladder. Collect bladder urine through the open drainage stopcock. Label this specimen "CB" (catheterized bladder urine) and refrigerate it.

3. Wash the bladder with 2 to 3 liters of sterile irrigating fluid.

4. When the bladder is empty, pass size 5 French polyethylene ureteral catheters through the cystoscope and into the bladder.

5. Introduce about 100 ml of irrigating fluid. Close the stopcock and drain the fluid from the bladder through the ureteral catheters. Collect a sample for culture and label it "WB" (washed bladder).

6. Pass each ureteral catheter to the middle or upper portion of each ureter.

7. Discard the first 5 to 10 ml of urine. Thereafter, collect 5 to 10 ml from each ureter in sterile tubes and label the tubes "LK" and "RK" (left kidney and right kidney) and "1," "2," or "3," indicating the sequence of collection. Refrigerate the tubes.

8. Transport all specimens to the laboratory for culture.

9. Pediatric needs: Same as for adults.

## Suprapubic Aspirate for Urine Cultures

A. Selection
  1. This technique avoids contamination of urine with urethral or perineal bacteria.
  2. The method is required for diagnosing anaerobic urinary tract infections and is most frequently used for pediatric patients, patients with a spinal cord injury, and patients for whom a definitive culture has not been obtained.

B. Collection
  1. Materials
    a. Supplies for skin decontamination
    b. Local anesthetic
    c. 22-gauge needle and syringe
    d. Sterile urine container
  2. Method
    a. Decontaminate the skin from the umbilicus to the urethra. Anesthetize the skin at the insertion site.
    b. Introduce the needle into the full bladder at the midline between the symphysis pubis and the umbilicus, 2 cm above the symphysis.
    c. Aspirate about 20 ml of urine from the bladder.
    d. Transfer the urine aseptically into a sterile screw-cap cup for transport to the laboratory.

C. Labeling
  1. Label the specimen with patient information, including the patient's age.
  2. Indicate on the request form that the specimen is a urine aspirate.
  3. Indicate whether or not anaerobic studies are required.
  4. Indicate the time of collection.

D. Transport
  1. If the specimen will not be transported to the laboratory within 30 min of collection, refrigerate it.
  2. If no one is in the laboratory to receive the specimen, place it in the laboratory refrigerator.

**E.** Comments
  1. Anaerobic studies are done only on request.
  2. Pediatric needs: This procedure can be used on infants to confirm the positive results obtained from a strapped-on bag device; however, thorough cleansing is mandatory, especially with pediatric patients who are diapered and may have larger amounts of skin and fecal flora on the skin in the diaper area. The insertion site is usually 1 to 2 cm above the pubic symphysis on the abdomen. After occlusion of the urethral opening to prevent leakage of urine, the skin is punctured. When the needle enters the bladder cavity, a small amount of urine is aspirated. Five milliliters of urine or less is adequate for culture in this population. If the bladder is partially empty, however, this angle may cause the needle to pass over the top of the bladder, resulting in an unsuccessful aspiration.

## ▨ Urine Specimens: Bladder Washout

Bladder washout, although seldom used, can assist in determining whether a bladder infection or a kidney infection exists. In principle, the bladder is rinsed via a urethral catheter to eliminate bacteria. Specimens are then obtained from the catheter and cultured quantitatively. Later specimens should represent urine from the kidney without contamination from organisms previously located in the bladder. If the kidney is involved, the post-bladder rinse should contain large numbers of organisms, whereas in bladder infections, this specimen shows no growth.

1. Insert an indwelling catheter into the bladder.

2. Save the last portion of the urine flow for culture. Refrigerate it immediately.

3. Introduce a specified volume of a solution of neomycin (0.1 to 0.2%). Some clinicians add elastase (a mixture of bovine fibrinolysin and DNase) to the solution. Allow the solution to remain in the bladder for 30 min.

4. Wash the bladder with 2 liters of sterile irrigating fluid and drain the bladder.

5. Collect three samples at 10-min intervals. Label the initial and subsequent timed collections.

6. Pediatric needs: Same as for adults. In an emergency situation, a wash with several milliliters of sterile nonbacteriostatic saline may aid in the diagnosis of a bladder infection in children who are unable to produce adequate amounts of urine for culture.

## ▨ Urine Specimens: Ileal Conduit

An ileal conduit uses a segment of ileum as a replacement for another tubular organ, such as in the formation of an artificial bladder into which ureters can be implanted following a total cystectomy. The proximal end of the ileal segment is closed, and the distal opening is brought to skin level as a stoma. Urine is collected in an ileostomy bag.

1. Remove the urinary appliance and discard the contained urine (which is not suitable for culture).

2. Swab the stomal opening with an alcohol wipe or iodine compound.

3. Aseptically insert a sterile no. 14 Robnel catheter (or a no. 10 or no. 12 Robnel catheter for ureterostomies) into the stoma and catheterize the ileal conduit to a depth beyond the fascial level.

4. Collect the urine drained from the catheter in a sterile container and either transport it directly to the laboratory or refrigerate it.

5. Pediatric needs: Same as for adults except for catheter size.

## *Chlamydia* Culture

Table 15 lists collection methods for specimens for *Chlamydia* testing.

When specimens are collected for enzyme immunoassay or other antigen detection methods, follow the manufacturer's instructions and use the swabs provided. Some swabs may not be satisfactory. As a general rule, do not use swabs with wooden sticks. Cytobrush specimens may be more productive than swab samples.

Special *Chlamydia* transport medium is essential to successful culture. Urine can be useful for some nonculture tests for men but not for women, so follow the manufacturer's instructions. Keep the specimen cold and transport it rapidly to the laboratory.

**Table 15** Specimens and collection methods for *Chlamydia* testing

| Specimen | Collection |
| --- | --- |
| For direct examination | Scrape the site with a swab and roll the swab (method of choice) onto the slide provided. Organisms are found inside epithelial cells. |
| For culture<br>    Cervix | *Chlamydia* infects the columnar and squamocolumnar cells; therefore, it is necessary to swab the endocervical canal area (the transitional zone or the os) vigorously to obtain cells. Place the swab in *Chlamydia* transport medium and vigorously agitate it to remove the contents. Discard the swab. Freeze at –70°C within 24 h and hold at 4°C until frozen. The use of a cytobrush is also effective. |
|     Eye | Do not sample exudate; remove it. Swab conjunctiva as firmly as possible. |
|     Lymph node aspirate | Place in an equal volume of transport medium. |
|     Nasopharyngeal aspirate | Place in an equal volume of transport medium. |
|     Sputum | Place in an equal volume of transport medium. |
|     Tissue | Place in an equal volume of transport medium. |
|     Urethra | Insert swab 4 to 6 cm into the urethra and rotate it to obtain epithelial cells. Remove the swab, place it in *Chlamydia* transport medium, and vigorously agitate it to remove its contents. Discard the swab. |
|     Cytology | Air-dry smears or scrapings. Fix in acetone or methanol for fluorescent antibody staining or fix in methanol for Giemsa staining. Heat for Macchiavello or Gimenez staining. |

**131**

Pediatric needs: Same as for adults. A sterile swab can be used to obtain conjunctival or nasopharyngeal specimens for culture in neonates or for a vaginal (girls) or urethral (boys) culture in prepubescent children. A swab can also be used for collection of genital specimens from adolescents that will be tested by a method that detects *Chlamydia* antigen. At this time, only confirmation of infection by culture may be acceptable as evidence concerning legal issues of sexual abuse in prepubescent children. Check the state laws.

## Specimens for *Mycoplasma* and *Ureaplasma* spp.

Specimens for the detection of *Mycoplasma* spp. are usually of respiratory or urogenital origin, although other specimens such as blood and other body fluids can be submitted. Samples from carefully taken throat swabs and early-morning sputum specimens are both valuable for detection of this organism in the respiratory tract. It is important for throat specimens that the affected area be firmly sampled to obtain mucosal cells. The swab is first immersed and agitated in transport medium; then the fluid is expressed from the swab and the swab is removed and discarded prior to transport. Specimens can be transported and stored in mycoplasma growth medium, nutrient broth enriched with serum, or sucrose-phosphate transport medium (2SP). The 2SP medium can also be used for transport of specimens for isolation of *Chlamydia*. Specimens can be held at 4°C for up to 24 h, although ideally specimens should be cultured within 6 h. Long-term storage should be at –70°C.

Both *Ureaplasma and Mycoplasma* spp. can be isolated from the urogenital tract. For males, urethral swabs are commonly used. Vaginal, cervical, or urethral swabs from women can be submitted, although mollicutes are not usually associated with vaginitis. Urine also can be submitted for analysis but yields fewer organisms than swab specimens. Transport and storage conditions are the same as for respiratory specimens.

## Fungal Specimens

A. Selection
  1. Specimens for fungal culture are collected as described for bacterial culture for:
  Wounds and abscesses
  Blood (Special bottles or the lysis centrifugation method can be used. Consult the laboratory.)
  Body fluids (up to 50 ml; never on swabs)
  Skin ulcers (Punch biopsy of active margin. Swab periphery and base of suspected sporothrix lesion.)
  Sputum
  Tissue
  Urine
  Genitals
  2. Select affected hair, skin, and nails for laboratory evaluation.
  3. Mucous membranes of the mouth and vagina can be scraped with a tongue depressor. Submit material in saline.

B. Collection
  1. Materials
     a. Forceps
     b. Scalpel
     c. 70% alcohol for disinfection
     d. Sterile tube or clean envelope
     e. Gauze
     f. Wood's lamp
  2. Method
     a. Hair. Remove at least 10 to 12 affected hairs with forceps. Place them in a clean tube or small envelope. Do not use stopper tubes because moisture accumulation may contaminate the specimen. Select the hairs that fluoresce under a Wood's lamp.
     b. Skin. Clean the skin surface with 70% alcohol. Scrape the surface of the skin at the *active margin* of the lesion and remove superficial material. Do not draw blood when scraping the skin. Place the scraping in a clean envelope or glass tube or between two glass slides which should then be taped together.

    c. Nails. Remove nail polish from the nail to be sampled. Wipe the nail with 70% alcohol on gauze (not cotton). Collect debris from *under* the nail and place it in a clean envelope or glass tube. Scrape the *outer* surface of the nail and discard the scraping. Collect scrapings from the deeper, diseased areas of the nail and add them to the material previously collected from under the nail. Nail clippings may also be submitted.

C. Labeling
1. Label the specimen with patient information.
2. Identify the specimen source clearly.
3. Note the suspected diagnosis if possible.
4. Ensure that the envelopes are sealed.

D. Transport
1. Do *not* refrigerate the specimen. Submit it at room temperature.

E. Comments
1. Culture for fungi may take several weeks because fungi grow slowly. Results from staining are available sooner. Some specimens may be placed directly into dermatophyte medium.
2. For systemic infections, consider the need for acute- and convalescent-phase sera.
3. Always sample the periphery (advancing margin) of a skin lesion.
4. Keep biopsy material moist by placing it between pieces of sterile, moistened gauze in a small dish.
5. Swabs are usually *not* recommended for collecting fungal specimens except when used to swab the vagina for yeasts or to swab sporotrichotic chancres.
6. Pediatric needs: Same as for adults.

*We can have the highest-skilled technologists using the most sensitive and sophisticated assays, but we can't make up for a poor specimen.*
WALLACE H. GREENE, Ph.D., ABMM
M. S. Hershey Medical Center, Hershey, PA

## Rickettsial Specimens
### (Rocky Mountain spotted fever)

Generally, rickettsial disease is diagnosed clinically, but it can be diagnosed in the clinical laboratory by direct detection of rickettsiae in patient tissues, isolation of the agent from tissues, and serologic testing for rickettsial antibodies (33). In most cases, serodiagnosis with an acute-phase serum sample (obtained early in the disease) and a convalescent-phase serum sample (obtained 1 to 3 weeks later) is the best approach.

The method of choice is fluorescence microscopy. For a biopsy, locate a macule or petechia and place a small, 1-mm-thick ink dot in its center. Obtain a full-thickness, 3-mm-diameter punch biopsy sample that encompasses the entire ink mark and *includes the dermis.* Freeze the sample on dry ice in a sealed container.

*Culture of these organisms represents a significant safety hazard and should be done only by reference laboratories.*

Pediatric needs: Same as for adults.

## Viral Specimens

Appropriate preanalytical specimen management practices have a profound effect on the outcome of laboratory analysis for viral diseases. For example, manufacturers of viral transport media provide components and instructions on how to use their device for specimen collection along with recommended transport time and temperature conditions. Table 16 lists collection methods for specimens for viral testing.

For in-house testing (those not being sent to an off-site laboratory), a transport time to the laboratory of <2 h is ideal and although most tests (except culture) will work well from specimens transported at ambient temperature, transport on ice or in a cold pack is often recommended by manufacturers. Specimens should not be frozen unless transport will take >24 h, at which point freezing at −60°C or −70°C or on dry ice is recommended, never at −20°C (23, 34); however, these temperatures may impact RSV, CMV, and VZV (35).

Sampling of patients should take into account the phase of disease. In addition, viral shedding depends upon the virus, the infected organ, and host responses:

- Prodrome – pre symptoms – shedding may begin here
- Acute phase – shedding decreases; IgM appears
- Resolution phase – shedding stops; IgG appears

Occasionally new or novel viruses appear, often as a public health concern. During these events, there is often a lack of information or consensus on how to obtain a laboratory diagnosis in the community hospital. The local or state public health laboratory should be consulted during these events to obtain guidance on specimen management activities. In addition, the CDC will be a leader and source of validated information related to an emerging viral disease. The most recent example would be the emergence of Zika virus and its devastating impact on the developing fetus. Refer to the CDC or other regulatory website for the most current specimen collection and testing guidelines.

Transport conditions are critical and virus viability may be impacted by inappropriate conditions (34). For example:

- RSV is thermolabile: there is approximately a 90% loss of infectivity after 24 h at 37°C and 4 d at 4°C (36).
- Adenovirus is stable in M4RT for 5 d at ambient temp (37).
- Prompt delivery is ideally 1 h after collection; however, a 2 h transport time is likely acceptable.
- Transportation of most specimens is acceptable at RT or 4°C (ice/cold pack), except for blood and CSF, which should be transported at RT.

**Table 16** Specimens and collection methods for viral testing

| Specimen | Collection method |
| --- | --- |
| Bronchoalveolar lavage | Flexible fiber-optic bronchoscope, as for bacterial culture |
| Cervix | Place swab into endocervix and rotate it gently for 10 s |
| Eye (conjunctiva, cornea) | As for bacteria |
| Gastrointestinal (feces, rectal swab contents) | As for bacteria |
| Genital lesion | Collect vesicle fluid with a tuberculin syringe and a 26-gauge needle, bevel side up, or unroof a fresh vesicle and vigorously scrape the base of the lesion with a swab or scalpel blade. Old vesicles do not contain virus. |
| Nasal washing | Use a 1-oz rubber suction bulb with 3 to 7 ml of phosphate-buffered saline. Tilt the patient's head back to a 70° angle and squeeze and release the bulb once. A flocked swab specimen from the nares may be equally effective. |
| Nasopharyngeal | Collect on a calcium alginate swab as for bacteria. Place in viral transport medium. |
| Skin lesion | Collect vesicle fluid with a tuberculin syringe and a 26-gauge needle, bevel side up, or unroof a fresh vesicle and vigorously scrape the base of the lesion with a swab or scalpel blade. Old vesicles do not contain virus. |
| Sputum | As for bacteria; not a specimen of choice |
| Throat | Collect as for bacteria or use a swab and viral transport medium. Patient can also gargle virus transport medium for 5 s and expectorate into a cup. |
| Urine | Collect two or three early-morning specimens as for bacteria. |
| Vagina | Place swab in vagina and firmly swab vaginal walls. |
| Blood | Collect 5 ml in a heparinized tube; separate lymphocytes and polymorphonuclear leukocytes. For serology, acute- and convalescent-phase sera are required. |
| Tissue | As for bacteria |

Pediatric needs: Specimens appropriate for testing for viral infection in pediatric populations include nasal washes and aspirates, contents of nasopharyngeal swabs, tracheal aspirates, and bronchoalveolar lavage, cerebrospinal fluid, feces or material from rectal swabs, urine, blood, tissue, and specimens from cutaneous eruptions such as vesicles. Swab specimens or material from small biopsies must be placed in viral transport medium, which is kept on ice for transport to the laboratory. Larger pieces of tissue or fluid specimens can be sent in a sterile container.

Testing of blood for the presence of viruses usually involves extraction of the buffy coat and culture of the leukocytes. Because of the relatively short period of viremia in healthy hosts, viral cultures of blood are usually the most beneficial in immunosuppressed patients. Since children undergoing transplantation or treatment of oncologic problems are often neutropenic and volumes of blood less than 2 ml are often received for testing, leukocyte extraction methods that optimize the concentration of cells in the buffy coat are required.

*Our virus isolation rate doubles whenever a physician or nurse calls for specimen collection information.*

C. GEORGE RAY, M.D.
St. Louis University Medical Center, St. Louis, MO

# WOUND SPECIMENS

## General Information

**A.** General terms like "*wound*," "*eye*," and "*ear*" are inappropriate for describing a specimen source. The name of a specific anatomic site is required.

**B.** The requisition should distinguish between surface wounds and deep or surgical wounds (Fig. 28). Material from surface wounds is not cultured for anaerobes, but that from deep wounds is.

**C.** Attention to skin decontamination is critical.

**D.** The quality of a wound culture should be assessed by Gram staining. The presence of epithelial cells indicates contamination with skin flora and may invalidate the significance of culture results. Many microbiologists are reluctant to do anaerobic bacteriology procedures on wound specimens containing small numbers of squamous epithelial cells (e.g., about five) per a 100× magnification field (2, 25).

**E.** The representative specimen is taken from the advancing margin of the lesion and is *not* just pus or exudate. It is critical that lesion margins and abscess walls be firmly sampled with a swab (3).

**Figure 28** Wound specimens should, at the least, be labeled as "surface wound" or "deep wound." The laboratory depends on this information for selecting appropriate culture media and interpreting results.

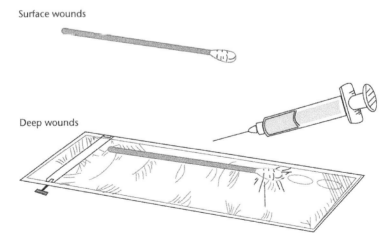

F. For anaerobic studies, the specimen of choice is an aspirate, not a swab. Anaerobic transport media must be used when requests for anaerobic culture are submitted. Anaerobes cannot survive in the presence of air.

G. Follow the manufacturer's instructions regarding the type of swab to be used with a specific FDA-cleared test product.

## ▨ Ear (Otitis Media) Specimens

**A.** Selection
  1. Since the infection is behind the tympanum, a swab is *not* recommended for collecting specimens used in the diagnosis of otitis media infections. When a swab is used, external ear canal flora contaminates the specimen, making interpretation of clinically relevant growth difficult and misleading.
  2. The specimen of choice is an aspirate from behind the tympanum (ear drum) (Fig. 29). The fluid from the inner ear represents the infectious process, not the external ear canal flora.
  3. A small swab may be used only when the ear drum has ruptured and fluid can be collected. First clean the external ear canal.
  4. Diagnosis of otitis media is usually made clinically. Tympanocentesis is painful and is performed only on young children and on patients with chronic otitis media that does not respond to therapy.

**Figure 29**  Diagram of the ear. A swab is not the specimen of choice for laboratory diagnosis of otitis media because it obviously will not reach the infected area. Preparing the ear for specimen collection is a critical step in obtaining an appropriate specimen.

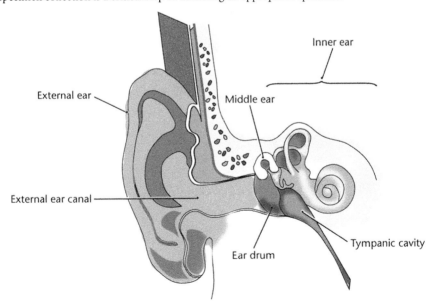

**B.** Collection
1. Materials
   a. Myringotome
   b. Ear speculum
   c. Ear forceps
   d. Suction device (syringe and needle)
   e. Anesthesia equipment
   f. Swabs and antiseptic
2. Method (tympanocentesis)
   a. Clean the external ear canal with antiseptic solution. After initial cleaning, antiseptic gauze can be packed into the ear until the physician is ready to proceed.
   b. The patient can be given a general anesthetic since the incision causes great pain.
   c. The physician surgically incises the ear drum and collects as much fluid as possible in a drainage tube. Alternatively, a 1-ml tuberculin syringe fitted with a 3.5-in 22-gauge spinal needle bent at a 30° angle can be inserted through the tympanum to aspirate fluid. Material from the drainage can also be allowed to collect on a sterile swab. The ear speculum helps prevent contamination by ear canal flora.
   d. Material in the syringe or drainage tubing can be aspirated into an anaerobic transport vial or submitted directly in the capped syringe.

**C.** Labeling
1. Do *not* label the specimen "*ear.*" If fluid has been collected, it should be appropriately labeled as "*tympanocentesis fluid.*"
2. Provide patient information.
3. Indicate the age of the patient and any pertinent history, e.g., "chronic otitis not responding to therapy."
4. Do not request anaerobic culture unless an anaerobic transport method is used.

**D.** Transport
1. Do *not* refrigerate the specimen.
2. Transport the specimen to the laboratory quickly. Hold it at room temperature.

**E.** Comments

1. Sample external ear infections (otitis externa) after cleaning the ear canal with a disinfectant and rinsing it with saline. Sample the canal several minutes after cleansing by swabbing briskly over any lesions present.

2. Tympanocentesis is infrequently performed, but it is the method of choice for obtaining specimens for culture.

3. Pediatric needs: Otitis is common in children of preschool age. Tympanocentesis is the specimen collection method of choice. If a myringotomy is done, fluid retrieved from the drainage tubing can be collected in a sterile vial or syringe for transport to the laboratory.

## Eye Specimens

A. Selection

1. Do not use the term "*eye*" in identifying a specimen. Specify what the specimen is, e.g., lid margin sample, conjunctival sample, corneal sample, aqueous or vitreous sample (Fig. 30). Specify left or right eye.
2. In serious eye infections, such as suppurative keratitis and endophthalmitis, the physician and the microbiologist must communicate so that appropriate media and transport systems are made available. For bacteria, chocolate agar is usually a good universal medium.
3. The method of specimen collection depends on the site of the eye infection (see below). In bilateral conjunctivitis, culture of a specimen from only one eye is necessary.
4. For conjunctival specimens, the laboratory ideally needs two swabs from the infected site: one for culture and one for Gram staining. Better Gram stain results are obtained with scrapings, not swab specimens, from the lid margin, conjunctiva, or cornea.

B. Collection

1. Materials
   a. Sterile Kimura spatula or an instrument for scraping
   b. Sterile calcium alginate swabs, two per package
   c. Sterile cotton swabs, two per package
   d. Frosted, etched-glass slides
   e. Microslide holders

**Figure 30** Diagram of the eye. The nature and potential severity of infections of the eye dictate special attention to the details of specimen management and an accurate description of the specimen submitted for analysis.

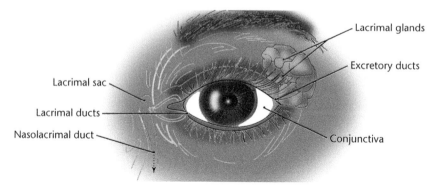

f.  Alcohol wipes

g.  Preservative-free, unit-dose 0.5% tetracaine

h.  Pencil or marker for labeling

2. Methods

a.  Methods are given in Table 17. For more detailed microbiology, refer to Cumitech 13B (38).

**Table 17**  Methods of collecting specimens from the eye

| Diagnosis | Specimen source | Method |
| --- | --- | --- |
| Preseptal cellulitis | Abscess drainage | For a *closed abscess*, prepare the skin for puncture. For *upper lid* suppuration, make an incision beneath the brow at the junction of the lateral one-third and medial two-thirds of the lid. For a lower lid abscess, make an incision at the site of maximum fluctuation, 1–2 cm above the inferior orbital rim. For an *open wound* or *drain site*, clean the adjacent skin thoroughly. The use of a needle and syringe is often not necessary. Submit drainage in an anaerobic transport vial. |
| Acute orbital cellulitis | Abscess drainage (biopsy) | Diagnosis is aided by an X-ray and a CAT[a] scan of the orbit and the paranasal sinuses. For an *open wound* or a *drain site*, aspirate with a needle and syringe. Submit specimen in the syringe or in an anaerobic transport vial. Use the method for a subperiosteal abscess, an intraorbital abscess, or an infected paranasal sinus. Sinus aspirate may reveal the etiologic agent of orbital cellulitis. |
| Canaliculitis | Canalicular material | Express purulent material by compressing the lid and canaliculus. Gram staining of this material may reveal typical bacterial morphology such as that of *Actinomyces* spp. A Kimura spatula can be used to transfer material to a culture medium. |
| Acute dacryocystitis | Conjunctiva | Transcutaneous aspiration or incision through the wall of the lacrimal sac may produce a fistula but relieves pressure in the sac and provides material for culture. The fistula will resolve once a dacryocystorhinostomy is performed. Moisten a swab with broth and obtain a conjunctival specimen. Aspirate drainage material from the lacrimal sac with a syringe and needle. |

*(Table continues on next page)*

**Table 17**  Methods of collecting specimens from the eye *(continued)*

| Diagnosis | Specimen source | Method |
|-----------|-----------------|--------|
| Blepharitis | Lid margin | Viral: There may not be enough fluid for needle aspiration. Culture a sample from a vesicle for the viral agent or submit it for immunofluorescence studies. <br> Bacterial: Scrub a cotton or calcium alginate swab moistened with the patient's tears or with broth across the anterior lid margins and ulcerated areas of the upper and lower lids of the right eye. Inoculate the lid margin specimens onto blood and chocolate agar in the shape of an R or an L, depending if the right or left eye was sampled. If both eyes are infected, the etiology is probably the same. Above the R or L on the chocolate plate, indicate conjunctiva with a vertical or horizontal streak of inoculum from the swab. Predominant growth may indicate the infection source as the conjunctiva or lid margin. |
| Conjunctivitis | Conjunctiva | Obtain specimens before instillation of a topical anesthetic. Moisten a cotton or calcium alginate swab with broth (unless exudate is present) and scrub it over the inferior tarsal conjunctiva and fornix of the infected eye. An additional swab can be taken for Gram staining. Use viral or bacterial transport as per request. |
| Keratitis | Cornea | Do not submit a corneal smear or anterior chamber fluid on a swab. Take conjunctival specimens with a calcium alginate swab and make a single row of C-shaped streaks on a chocolate agar. The second swab is used for a fungal medium if fungi are suspected. <br> Scrape a corneal ulcer with a spatula or a no. 15 blade scalpel. After anesthesia, scrape the cooled spatula over the surface of the area of suppuration in short, moderately firm strokes in one direction without touching the lashes or lids. Use each scraping to inoculate another row of C shapes on a chocolate plate or to make a smear. For viral keratitis, conjunctival exudate and scrapings in a viral transport vial are required. Virus is usually shed into the tears of the cul-de-sac, making conjunctival viral culture useful. |

| Endophthalmitis | Wound abscess, fistula, intraocular fluid, conjunctiva (to assess contamination of other sources) | Conjunctival cultures may provide minimal clinically relevant information if used alone. Sampling a purulent wound abscess may be helpful, but the most useful information may come from an aspirate of intraocular fluid from the patient in the operating room. |
|---|---|---|
| | | Obtain anterior chamber and vitreous fluid. Collect 1–2 ml of vitreous fluid by needle aspiration or, ideally, vitrectomy. Medium should be available at the bedside. |

*CAT, computed axial tomography.*

C. Labeling
1. Label the specimen with the actual diagnosis, not with the word "*eye.*"
2. Label the specimen as being from the right or the left eye.
3. Label the specimen with patient information.

D. Transport
1. Many specimens should be plated at the specimen collection site, e.g., the eye clinic. The small amount of material collected tends to dry quickly, and this drying may contribute to a loss of viability of test agents.
2. Use anaerobic transport where necessary but *not* for conjunctival specimens.
3. Chill the viral transport medium for transport.
4. Pediatric needs: Same as for adults.

## ▩ Skin and Contiguous Tissue Specimens (Wound, Abscess, Burn, Exudate)

A. Selection
   1. The specimen of choice depends on the extent and character of the infection rather than on the suspected pathogen.
   2. For most open lesions, remove the superficial flora *before* collecting a specimen by firmly sampling from the advancing margin or base.
   3. For dry, encrusted lesions, culture is not recommended unless an exudate is present.
   4. A closed abscess is the specimen site of choice. Collect exudate *and* a sample of the abscess wall.
   5. For an open abscess, decontaminate the lesion first, as for other open lesions.
   6. Culture burn wounds only after extensive cleaning and debridement. Biopsy specimens are recommended. Quantitative culture of burn surfaces may or may not be of value.
   7. The specimen of choice is taken from the advancing margin or base of the lesion and is not just pus. Remove the exudate to reach to the interior of the lesion.

B. Collection
   1. Material
      a. Skin disinfectant
      b. Sterile swabs
      c. Syringe and needle
      d. Anaerobic or aerobic transport medium
   2. Method
      a. Unruptured abscess. Do *not* swab. Decontaminate the skin overlying the abscess and aspirate the abscess contents with a syringe. After excision and draining, submit a portion of the abscess wall for culture. Submit the specimen in an anaerobic transport container.
      b. Open lesions and abscesses. Remove as much of the superficial flora as possible by decontaminating the skin. Remove exudate and firmly sample the base or margin of the lesion with a swab. Submit the swab in aerobic transport medium. You can also culture a sample of the exudate aerobically. Do not request anaerobic cultures of material from open superficial lesions. Consult with the laboratory.

    c. Burn wounds. Debride the area and disinfect the wound. As exudate appears, sample it firmly with a swab. Submit the sample for aerobic culture only. Submit biopsy tissue as the specimen of choice. Surface specimens usually represent colonization.

    d. Pustules or vesicles. Select an intact pustule. Apply alcohol and allow it to dry. Unroof the pustule with a 23-gauge needle (for pediatric patients). Collect fluid and basal cells by rotating the swab vigorously in the pustule. If the pustule is large, an 18-gauge needle on a tuberculin syringe can be used to puncture it. If the lesion is older, the crust should be removed and the moist base of the lesion sampled by swabbing with a premoistened sterile swab.

    e. Petechiae, purpura, or ecthyma gangrenosa. Collect specimen by vigorous scraping of the outer margin of the lesion.

    f. Scabies. This is usually a clinical diagnosis, and specimens for microbiology may not be indicated, although scrapings of infected skin may be requested.

**C.** Labeling
1. Do *not* label the specimen only as "*wound*" without giving a specific description and the anatomic source.
2. Label the specimen with patient information.
3. Note whether the exudate is from an open or a closed wound.
4. Indicate aerobic or anaerobic culture requests.
    a. Aerobic only. Submit in aerobic transport medium.
       i. Superficial-lesion exudates
       ii. Open-wound exudates
       iii. Laceration exudates
       iv. Open-abscess exudates
    b. Anaerobe and aerobe requests. Submit in anaerobic transport medium.
       i. Surgical aspirates
       ii. Closed-abscess aspirates
       iii. Biopsy tissue

**D.** Transport
1. Transport the specimen to the laboratory quickly.
2. Refrigerate the specimen if it will not be cultured within 1 h.

**E.** Comments
1. Skin decontamination is critical to proper culture interpretation.

2. The laboratory evaluates specimens by Gram staining. The presence of epithelial cells in the smear indicates surface contamination, and the results of culture will be compromised. The presence of leukocytes in the absence of epithelial cells represents an appropriate specimen.
3. Do *not* submit only pus. Pus is not a representative specimen of the lesion. Sample the advancing margin or base of the lesion.
4. Pediatric needs: Pediatric infections are often accompanied by skin eruptions such as rashes or vesicle formation. These specimen sites must be carefully cultured in order to optimize retrieval of pathogens. Wound specimens in which no inflammatory cells are present may be representative of superficial flora unrelated to the disease process and should be recollected.

*If there is a clinical issue, forget the swab and get some tissue.*

MICHAEL SAUBOLLE, Ph.D.
Banner Health, Phoenix, AZ

# SECTION IV Specimen Management Summary Tables

*The tables that follow summarize and document the salient features of the common specimens that arrive in the microbiology laboratory. The literature supporting these guidelines is included in case further study is warranted. Ensure laboratory safety procedures are in place and understood by everyone handling specimens (12).*

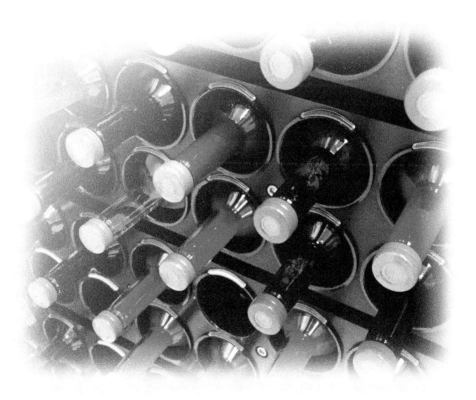

**Table 18** Bacteriology and mycology specimen collection guidelines[a]

| Specimen type (reference[s]) | Collection | | Time and temp | | Replica limits | Comment(s) |
|---|---|---|---|---|---|---|
| | Guidelines | Device and/or minimum vol | Local transport[b] | Courier or local storage | | |
| Abscess (2, 3, 13, 25) | Remove surface exudate by wiping with sterile saline or 70% EtOH. | | | | | More detail for fungal specimen management is found in reference (43). Tissue or fluid is always superior to a swab specimen. If swabs must be used, collect two, one for culture and one for Gram staining. Preserve and transport them with Stuart's or Amies medium. |
| Open | Aspirate, if possible, or pass a swab deep into the lesion and firmly sample the lesion's advancing edge. | Swab transport system | ≤2 h, RT | ≤24 h, RT | 1/day/source | A sample from the base of the lesion and a sample from the abscess wall are most productive. |
| Closed | Aspirate abscess wall material with needle and syringe. Aseptically transfer *all* material into anaerobic transport device. | Anaerobic transport system, ≥1 ml | ≤2 h, RT | ≤24 h, RT | 1/day/source | Sampling of the surface area can introduce colonizing bacteria not involved in the infectious process. |
| Bite wound (13, 44, 45) | See Abscess. | | | | | Do not culture animal bite wounds ≤12 h old (agents are usually not recovered) unless they are on the face or hand or unless signs of infection are present. |

*(Table continues on next page)*

155

**Table 18** Bacteriology and mycology specimen collection guidelines[a] *(continued)*

| Specimen type (reference[s]) | Collection | | Time and temp | | Replica limits | Comment(s) |
|---|---|---|---|---|---|---|
| | **Guidelines** | **Device and/or minimum vol** | **Local transport**[b] | **Courier or local storage** | | More detail for fungal specimen management is found in reference (43). |
| Blood cultures (27, 41, 46–50) | Disinfection of culture bottle: Apply 70% isopropyl alcohol to rubber stoppers and wait 1 min. Palpate for the vein first. Disinfect venipuncture site. Use commercial prep set with chlorhexidine or use protocol below: 1. Cleanse site with 70% alcohol. 2. Starting at the center, swab concentrically with an iodine preparation. 3. Allow the iodine to dry. 4. *Do not palpate the vein at this point.* 5. Collect blood. 6. After venipuncture, remove iodine from the skin with alcohol. | Bacteria: blood culture vials Adult, 10–20 ml/ set Higher volume most productive Infant, 1–10 ml/ set Fungi: 1. Biphasic culture 2. Lysis centrifugation | ≤2 h, RT | ≤24 h, RT or per instructions | 3 sets in 24 h | Follow manufacturer volume recommendations. Acute sepsis: 2–3 sets from separate sites, all within 10 min Endocarditis, acute: 3 sets from 3 separate sites, over 1–2 h Endocarditis, subacute: 3 sets from 3 separate sites, taken ≥15 min apart; if negative at 24 h, obtain 3 more sets. Fever of unknown origin: 2–3 sets from separate sites ≥1 h apart; if negative at 24 h, obtain 2–3 more sets. Some sites have determined that an additional aerobic bottle or fungal bottle is more productive than an anaerobic bottle. Adult bottles can be used with pediatric patients and their smaller volume blood draws. When an i.v. line is in place, draw blood from below the line to prevent dilution from the line contents. Blood drawn from shunts and catheters is more likely to result in contamination due to difficulty in decontaminating these devices. Lysis centrifugation is critical for *H. capsulatum* and other dimorphic fungi (51). Requests for cultures of blood bank products can be reviewed in reference (50). |

| Specimen | Collection | Container | Transport time/temp | Transport time/temp | No. | Comments |
|---|---|---|---|---|---|---|
| Bone marrow | Prepare puncture site as for surgical incision. | Inoculate blood culture bottle or a lysis centrifugation tube | ≤24 h, RT if in culture bottle or tube | ≤24 h, RT | 1/day | Small volumes of bone marrow may be inoculated directly onto culture media or into broth. Lysis centrifugation is critical for *H. capsulatum* and other dimorphic fungi (51). |
| Burn | Clean and debride the wound prior to specimen collection. | Tissue placed in a screw-cap container Swab exudate | ≤2 h, RT | ≤24 h, RT | 1/day/source | Process for aerobic culture only. A 3- to 4-mm punch biopsy is optimum when quantitative cultures are ordered; however, quantitative culture may or may not be valuable. Surface cultures of burns may be misleading. |
| Catheter i.v (52–54) | 1. Cleanse the skin around the catheter site with alcohol. 2. Aseptically remove catheter and clip a 5-cm distal tip of the catheter directly into a sterile tube. 3. Transport directly to microbiology to prevent drying. | Sterile screw-cap tube or cup | ≤15 min, RT | ≤24 h, 4°C | None | Acceptable i.v. catheters for semiquantitative culture (Maki method): central, CVP, Hickman, Broviac, peripheral, arterial, umbilical, hyperalimentation, Swan-Ganz. i.v. catheter tips submitted for culture should always be accompanied by a venipuncture blood culture for comparison and interpretation of the catheter results. Reject: Not acceptable for culture |
| Foley (16) | Do *not* culture since growth represents distal urethral flora. | | | | | |

(*Table continues on next page*)

**Table 18** Bacteriology and mycology specimen collection guidelines[a] (*continued*)

| Specimen type (reference[s]) | Collection | | Time and temp | | Replica limits | Comment(s) |
|---|---|---|---|---|---|---|
| | Guidelines | Device and/or minimum vol | Local transport[b] | Courier or local storage | | |
| Cellulitis (13, 55, 56) | 1. Cleanse site by wiping with sterile saline or 70% alcohol. 2. Aspirate the area of maximum inflammation (commonly the center rather than the leading edge) with a fine needle and syringe. 3. Draw small amount of sterile saline into syringe and aspirate into sterile screw-cap tube. | Sterile tube (syringe transport not recommended) | ≤15 min, RT | ≤24 h, RT | None | More detail for fungal specimen management is found in reference (43). Yield of potential pathogens is only 25–35%. |
| CSF (57–59) | 1. Disinfect site with 2% iodine tincture or other surgical preparation set 2. Insert a needle with stylet at L3-L4, L4-L5, or L5-S1 interspace. 3. On reaching the sub-arachnoid space, remove the stylet and collect 1–2 ml of fluid in each of three leakproof tubes. | Sterile screw-cap tube Minimum amount required: bacteria, ≥1 ml; fungi, ≥2 ml; AFB, ≥2 ml; Virus, ≥1 ml | Bacteria: never refrigerate; ≤15 min, RT Virus: transport on ice; ≤15 min, 4°C | ≤24 h, RT ≤72 h, 4°C | None | Obtain blood cultures also. If only 1 tube of CSF is collected, it should be sub-mitted to microbiology first; otherwise submit tube 2. Aspirate of brain abscess or a biopsy may be necessary to detect anaerobic bacteria or parasites. |

| Decubitus ulcer (13) | See comment: A swab is not the specimen of choice.<br>1. Cleanse surface with sterile saline.<br>2. If a sample biopsy is not available, vigorously swab the base of the lesion.<br>3. Place the swab in appropriate transport system. | Swab transport (aerobic) or anaerobic system (for tissue) | ≤2 h, RT | ≤24 h, RT | 1/day/source | A decubitus swab provides little relevant clinical information; discourage the use of swabs for this specimen.<br>A tissue biopsy sample or a needle aspirate is the specimen of choice. |
| Dental culture: gingival, periodontal, periapical, Vincent's stomatitis | See comment:<br>1. Carefully cleanse gingival margin and supragingival tooth surface to remove saliva, debris, and plaque.<br>2. Using a periodontal scaler, carefully remove subgingival lesion material and transfer it to an anaerobic transport system.<br>3. Prepare smears for staining that have been collected in the same fashion. | Anaerobic transport system | ≤2 h, RT | ≤24 h, RT | 1/day | Periodontal lesions should be processed by laboratories equipped to provide specialized techniques for the detection and enumeration of specific agents. |

*(Table continues on next page)*

**Table 18** Bacteriology and mycology specimen collection guidelines[a] *(continued)*

| Specimen type (reference[s]) | Collection | | Time and temp | | Replica limits | Comment(s) More detail for fungal specimen management is found in reference (43). |
|---|---|---|---|---|---|---|
| | Guidelines | Device and/or minimum vol | Local transport[b] | Courier or local storage | | |
| Ear | | | | | | |
| Inner (60) | Tympanocentesis should be reserved for complicated, recurrent, or chronic persistent otitis media.<br>1. For an intact ear drum, clean the ear canal with soap solution and collect fluid via the syringe aspiration technique.<br>2. For a ruptured ear drum, collect fluid for culture on a flexible-shaft swab via an otoscope. Collect a second swab for Gram stain. | Sterile tube, swab transport medium, or anaerobic system | ≤2 h, RT | ≤24 h, RT | 1/day/source | Many cases of otitis media may not require culture and are treated empirically. Throat or nasopharyngeal cultures are not predictive of agents responsible for otitis media and should not be submitted for that purpose.<br>Specimens can also be collected by needle aspiration of furuncles or by surgical debridement. |
| Outer (60) | 1. Use a moistened swab to remove any debris or crust from the ear canal.<br>2. Obtain a sample by firmly rotating the swab in the outer canal.<br>Collect a second swab for Gram stain. | Swab transport | ≤2 h, RT | ≤24 h, 4°C | 1/day/source | For otitis externa, *vigorous* swabbing is required since surface swabbing may miss streptococcal cellulitis. |

| | | | | |
|---|---|---|---|---|
| **Eye** | | | | |
| Conjunctiva (38, 41, 61) | 1. Sample both eyes using separate swabs (premoistened with sterile saline) by rolling over each conjunctiva.<br>2. Inoculate media at time of collection.<br>3. Smear swabs onto 2 slides for staining. | Direct culture inoculation: BHI with blood, CHOC, and inhibitory mold agar | Plates: ≤15 min, RT<br>Swabs: ≤2 h, RT | ≤24 h, RT | None | If possible, sample both conjunctivae, even if only one is infected, to determine the indigenous microflora. The uninfected eye can serve as a control with which to compare the agents isolated from the infected eye.<br>Ensure appropriate labeling; the specimen labeled "eye" is not helpful. Specify conjunctival, corneal, vitreous, and right or left eye, etc. Obtain dual swabs, one for culture and one for smear preparation. |
| Corneal scrapings (38, 41, 61) | 1. Obtain conjunctival swab specimens as described above.<br>2. Instill 2 drops of local anesthetic.<br>3. Using a sterile spatula, scrape ulcers or lesions and inoculate scraping directly onto media.<br>4. Apply remaining material to 2 clean glass slides for staining. | | ≤15 min, RT | None | It is recommended that swabs for culture be taken prior to anesthetic application, whereas corneal scrapings can be obtained afterward. |
| Fluid or aspirates | Prepare eye for needle aspiration of fluid. | Sterile screw-cap tube or direct inoculate of small amount of fluid onto media | ≤15 min, RT | ≤24 h, RT | 1/day | Include fungal media. Anesthetics may be inhibitory to some etiologic agents. |

*(Table continues on next page)*

**Table 18** Bacteriology and mycology specimen collection guidelines[a] *(continued)*

| Specimen type (reference[s]) | Collection | | Time and temp | | Replica limits | Comment(s) |
|---|---|---|---|---|---|---|
| | Guidelines | Device and/or minimum vol | Local transport[b] | Courier or local storage | | |
| **Feces** | | | | | | More detail for fungal specimen management is found in reference (43). |
| Routine culture (62) | Pass directly into a clean, dry container. Transport the specimen to microbiology laboratory within 1 h of collection or transfer a visible portion on a swab to a transport system such as Stuart's or Amies. | Clean, leakproof, wide-mouth container or a swab transport system; ≥2 g | Unpreserved: ≤1 h, RT Swab transport system: ≤24 h, RT | ≤24 h, 4°C ≤48 h, RT or 4°C | 1/day | For best results, test patients with active diarrhea in the acute stage of illness. Formed stools are often unproductive. Do not perform routine stool cultures on patients whose length of stay was >3 days and the admitting diagnosis was not gastroenteritis. Culture and toxin tests for *C. difficile* should be considered in these cases. Swabs for routine pathogens are not recommended except in infants and in patients with active diarrhea (see "Rectal and Anal Swab Specimens"). |
| *C. difficile* (62–64) | Pass liquid or soft stool directly into a clean, dry container. Soft stool is defined as stool assuming the shape of its container. A swab specimen is not recommended for toxin testing. | Sterile, leakproof, wide-mouth container; ≥5 ml | ≤1 h, RT; 1–24 h, 4°C; >24 h, −20°C | 2 days, 4°C, for culture 3 days, 4°C, or longer at −70°C for toxin test | 1/2 days | Patients should be passing ≥5 liquid or soft stools per 24 h. Testing of formed or hard stool is often unproductive and may indicate only commensal carriage. Reject formed stools and swabs for *C. difficile* toxin testing. Freezing at −20°C facilitates rapid loss of cytotoxin activity. |
| *Escherichia coli* O157:H7 (62) Shiga toxin producer | Pass liquid or bloody stool into a clean, dry container | Sterile, leakproof, wide-mouth container or swab transport system; >2 ml | Unpreserved: ≤1 h, RT Swab transport system: ≤24 h, RT or 4°C | ≤24 h, 4°C ≤48 h, RT | 1/day | Bloody or liquid stools collected within 6 days of onset from patients with abdominal cramps have the highest yield. Other *E. coli* serotypes may produce Shiga toxin so the test of choice, either detecting toxin or the toxin-encoding gene, should be capable of identifying non-O157 toxin producers as well. |

| Specimen | Collection | Container | Transport | | Frequency | Comments |
|---|---|---|---|---|---|---|
| Leukocytes (65) Lactoferrin | Pass feces directly into a clean, dry container. Transport specimen to microbiology laboratory within 1 h of collection or transfer to ova and parasite transport system (10% formalin or PVA). | Sterile, leakproof, wide-mouth container or 10% formalin and/or PVA; >2 ml | Unpreserved: ≤1 h, RT Formalin/PVA | ≤24 h, 4°C Indefinite, RT | 1/day | Fecal leukocytes are commonly found in patients with shigellosis and salmonellosis (erythrocytes) and sometimes in amebiasis. Mononuclear cells are found in typhoid fever. This procedure is discouraged by some because it may provide results with little clinical value and can be misleading. A Gram stain or a simple methylene blue stain can be used to visualize leukocytes. Commercial detection methods are also available. Commercial lactoferrin tests are also available. |
| Rectal swab | 1. Carefully insert a swab ~1 in. beyond the anal sphincter. 2. Gently rotate the swab to sample the anal crypts. 3. Feces should be visible on the swab for detection of diarrheal pathogens. | Swab transport | ≤2 h, RT | ≤24 h, RT | 1/day | For most patients, a swab is not the specimen of choice. Reserved for detecting *Neisseria gonorrhoeae*, *Shigella* spp., *Campylobacter* spp., HSV, and anal carriage of group B *Streptococcus* spp. or for patients unable to pass a specimen. |
| Fistulas | See Abscess | | | | | |

(Table continues on next page)

**Table 18** Bacteriology and mycology specimen collection guidelines[a] (*continued*)

| Specimen type (reference[s]) | Collection | | Time and temp | | Replica limits | Comment(s) |
|---|---|---|---|---|---|---|
| | Guidelines | Device and/or minimum vol | Local transport[b] | Courier or local storage | | |
| Fluids: abdominal, amniotic, ascites, bile, joint, paracentesis, pericardial, peritoneal, pleural, synovial, thoracentesis | 1. Disinfect overlying skin with 2% iodine tincture or chlorhexidine. 2. Obtain specimen via percutaneous needle aspiration or surgery. 3. Transport specimen to laboratory immediately. 4. Always submit as much fluid as possible, *never* submit a swab dipped in fluid. | Blood culture bottle for bacteria and yeast or sterile screw-cap tube or anaerobic transport system Bacteria, ≥1 ml; fungi, ≥10 ml; mycobacteria, ≥10 ml | ≤15 min, RT | ≤24 h, RT Pericardial fluid and fluids for fungal cultures: ≤24 h, 4°C | None | More detail for fungal specimen management is found in reference (43). Amniotic and culdocentesis fluids should be transported in anaerobic system and need not be centrifuged prior to Gram staining. Other fluids are best examined by Gram staining of a cytocentrifuged preparation. See Table 7. |
| Gangrenous tissue | See Abscess | | | | | Discourage sampling of surface or superficial tissue; tissue biopsy or aspirates are preferred. |
| Gastric: wash or lavage (66) | Collect early in the morning before patients eat and while they are still in bed. 1. Introduce a nasogastric tube orally or nasally into the stomach. 2. Perform lavage with 25–50 ml of chilled, sterile, distilled water. 3. Recover sample and place it in a leakproof, sterile container. 4. Before removing the tube, release suction and clamp it. | Sterile, leakproof container | ≤15 min, RT, or neutralize within 1 h of collection | ≤24 h, 4°C or on ice | 1/day | The specimen must be processed promptly since mycobacteria die rapidly in gastric washings. Neutralize each 35–50 ml of gastric washing with 1.5 ml of 40% anhydrous $Na_2HPO_4$. |

| Specimen | Collection procedure | Transport device | Transport time/temp | Replicate limit | Comments |
|---|---|---|---|---|---|
| **Genital (female)** | | | | | |
| Amniotic (67) | 1. Aspirate via amniocentesis, cesarean section, or intrauterine catheter.<br>2. Transfer fluid to an anaerobic transport system. | Anaerobic transport system, ≥1 ml | ≤15 min, RT | ≤24 h, RT | None | Swabbing or aspiration of vaginal membrane is *not* acceptable because of the potential for culture contamination by commensal vaginal flora. |
| Bartholin | 1. Disinfect skin with an iodine preparation.<br>2. Aspirate fluid from ducts. | Anaerobic transport system, ≥1 ml | ≤2 h, RT | ≤24 h, RT | 1/day | |
| Cervical (26) | 1. Visualize the cervix using a speculum without lubricant.<br>2. Remove mucus and secretions from the cervix with a swab and discard the swab.<br>3. Firmly, yet gently, sample the endocervical canal with a newly obtained sterile swab. | Swab transport | ≤2 h, RT | ≤24 h, RT | 1/day | See information on virus and chlamydia collection and transport needs.<br>*Neisseria gonorrhoeae* is found in exudates, whereas chlamydiae infect specific cells. |
| Cul-de-sac | Submit aspirate or fluid. | Anaerobic transport system, >1 ml | ≤2 h, RT | ≤24 h, RT | 1/day | |
| Endometrial | 1. Collect transcervical aspirate via a telescoping catheter.<br>2. Transfer the entire amount to an anaerobic transport system. | Anaerobic transport system, ≥1 ml | ≤2 h, RT | ≤24 h, RT | 1/day | |

*(Table continues on next page)*

**Table 18** Bacteriology and mycology specimen collection guidelines[a] *(continued)*

| Specimen type (reference[s]) | Collection | | Time and temp | | Replica limits | Comment(s) |
|---|---|---|---|---|---|---|
| | Guidelines | Device and/or minimum vol | Local transport[b] | Courier or local storage | | More detail for fungal specimen management is found in reference (43). |
| Placenta | 1. Use a sterile swab to collect material from the carefully exposed chorion-amnion interface. 2. Place placenta fetal side up to begin procedure. 3. Culture site is at the base of the umbilicus. 4. Cut through the chorionic membrane exposing the chorion-amnion interface. 5. Firmly swab this interface and place swab into transport. | Swab or sterile screw-cap jar | ≤2 h, RT | ≤24 h, RT | 1/patient | The value of performing routine placental cultures appears limited. Placenta culture should only come from cesarean delivery. Positive or negative placental cultures are often not helpful even when histology suggests disease. The current method of placental swabbing and culture technique is highly specific but not sensitive. |
| Products of conception | 1. Submit a portion of tissue in a sterile container. 2. If obtained by cesarean section, immediately transfer it to an anaerobic transport system. | Sterile tube or anaerobic transport system | ≤2 h, RT | ≤24 h, RT | 1/day | Do not process lochia. Culture of this specimen may or may not provide clinically relevant results, and such results can be misleading. |
| Urethral (26) | Collect 1 h after patient has urinated. 1. Remove exudate from the urethral orifice. 2. Collect discharge material on a swab by massaging the urethra against the pubic symphysis through the vagina. | Swab transport | ≤2 h, RT | ≤24 h, RT | 1/day | If no discharge can be obtained, wash the external urethra with betadine soap and rinse with water. Insert a urethrogenital swab 2-4 cm into the urethra; rotate swab for 2 s. |

| Vaginal (26) | 1. Wipe away an excessive amount of secretion or discharge.<br>2. Obtain secretions from the mucosal membrane of the vaginal vault with a sterile swab or pipette.<br>3. If a smear is also requested, use a second swab. | Swab transport | ≤2 h, RT | ≤24 h, RT | 1/day | For intrauterine devices, place entire device in a sterile container and submit at RT.<br>Gram staining is recommended for confirmation of bacterial vaginosis. Results from cultures are often inaccurate and misleading. Commercial PCR instruments are also available and the manufacturer's instructions must be followed. |
| Genital (female or male)<br>Lesion (23) | 1. Clean the lesion with sterile saline and remove the surface of the lesion with a sterile scalpel blade.<br>2. Allow transudate to accumulate.<br>3. Pressing the base of the lesion, *firmly* sample exudate with a sterile swab. | Swab transport | ≤2 h, RT | ≤24 h, RT | 1/day | For dark-field examination to rule out syphilis, touch a glass slide to the transudate, add a coverslip, and transport immediately to the laboratory in a humidified chamber (petri dish with moist gauze).<br>Specimens for syphilis should not be submitted for culture.<br>DFA-*Treponema pallidum* is typically performed in public health laboratories and requires the same type specimen.<br>Treponemal and nontreponemal serology requires serum submitted in a clot tube at RT in <2 h after collection. Treponemal tests include TPPA and FTA-ABS that usually remain positive for life. |

*(Table continues on next page)*

**Table 18** Bacteriology and mycology specimen collection guidelines[a] *(continued)*

| Specimen type (reference[s]) | Collection | | Time and temp | | Replica limits | Comment(s) |
|---|---|---|---|---|---|---|
| | Guidelines | Device and/or minimum vol | Local transport[b] | Courier or local storage | | More detail for fungal specimen management is found in reference (43). |
| **Genital (male)** | | | | | | |
| Prostate (23, 68) | 1. Cleanse the glans with soap and water. 2. Massage the prostate through the rectum. 3. Collect fluid on a sterile swab or in a sterile tube. | Swab transport or sterile tube | ≤1 h, RT or 4°C | ≤24 h, RT | 1/day | More relevant results may be obtained by adding a urine specimen immediately before and after massage to indicate urethral and bladder organisms. Ejaculate can also be cultured. |
| Urethra | Insert a urethrogenital swab 2–4 cm into the urethral lumen, rotate the swab, and leave it in place for at least 2 s to facilitate absorption. | Swab transport | ≤2 h, RT | ≤24 h, RT | 1/day | |
| Hair: dermatophytosis (51, 69) | 1. With forceps, collect at least 10–12 affected hairs with the base of the shaft intact. Get the hair root if possible. Select hair strands that fluoresce with a Wood's lamp. 2. Place in a clean tube or container. | Clean container, 10 hairs | ≤24 h, RT | | 1/day/site | Collect scalp scales, if present, along with scrapings of active borders of lesions. Note any antifungal therapy taken recently. |

| Specimen | Collection procedure | Container | Transport | Storage | Frequency | Comments |
|---|---|---|---|---|---|---|
| Nail: dermatophytosis (51, 69) | 1. Wipe the nail with 70% alcohol using gauze (not cotton). 2. Clip away a generous portion of the affected area and collect material or debris from *under* the nail. 3. Place material in a clean container. | Clean container Need enough scrapings to cover the head of a thumb tack | ≤24 h, RT | | 1/day | Minced nail pieces will be pressed down into agar to facilitate recovery of dermatophytes. |
| Pilonidal cyst | See Abscess | | | | | |
| Respiratory, lower Bronchoalveolar lavage, bronchial brush or wash, tracheal aspirate | 1. Place aspirate or washing in a sputum trap. 2. Place brush in a sterile container with saline. | Sterile container, >1 ml | ≤2 h, RT | ≤24 h, 4°C | 1/day | 40–80 ml of fluid needed for quantitative analysis. For quantitative analysis of brushings, place brush in 0.5 ml of Trypticase soy broth for transport. |
| Sputum, expectorate (51, 70) | 1. Collect the specimen under the direct supervision of a nurse or physician. 2. Have the patient rinse or gargle with water to reduce superficial oral flora. Brushing teeth and tongue helps. 3. Instruct the patient to cough deeply to produce a lower respiratory tract specimen (not postnasal fluid). Collect in a sterile container. | Sterile container, >1 ml Minimum amounts: bacteria, >1 ml; fungi, 3–5 ml; mycobacteria, 5–10 ml; parasites, 3–5 ml | ≤2 h, RT | ≤24 h, 4°C | 1/day | In pediatric patients unable to produce a specimen, a respiratory therapist should collect a specimen via suction. The best specimen should have ≤10 squamous cells per 100× field. |

(Table continues on next page)

**Table 18** Bacteriology and mycology specimen collection guidelines[a] (continued)

| Specimen type (reference[s]) | Collection | | Time and temp | | Replica limits | Comment(s) |
|---|---|---|---|---|---|---|
| | Guidelines | Device and/or minimum vol | Local transport[b] | Courier or local storage | | More detail for fungal specimen management is found in reference (43). |
| Sputum, induced (70) | 1. Have the patient rinse the mouth with water after brushing the gums and tongue. 2. With the aid of a nebulizer, have the patient inhale ~25 ml of 3–10% saline. 3. Collect the induced sputum in a sterile container. | Sterile container | ≤2 h, RT | ≤24 h, RT | 1/day | *Histoplasma capsulatum* and *Blastomyces dermatitidis* survive for only short periods of time once a specimen is obtained. Fungal recovery is primarily for *Cryptococcus* spp. and some filamentous fungi; other yeasts rarely cause lower respiratory tract infection. Lysis with mucolytic agents followed by centrifugation facilitates detection of *Pneumocystis jirovecii* and other fungi. |
| Respiratory, upper (23) Oral | 1. Remove oral secretions and debris from the surface of the lesion with a swab and discard swab. 2. Using a second swab, vigorously sample the lesion, avoiding any areas of normal tissue. | Swab transport | ≤2 h, RT | ≤24 h, RT | 1/day | Discourage sampling of superficial tissue for bacterial evaluation. Tissue biopsy or needle aspirates are the specimens of choice. |
| Nasal | 1. Insert a swab, premoistened with sterile saline, ~2 cm into the nares. 2. Rotate the swab against the nasal mucosa. | Swab transport | ≤2 h, RT | ≤24 h, RT | 1/day | Anterior nose cultures should be reserved for detecting staphylococcal and streptococcal carriers or for nasal lesions. |
| Nasopharynx (23) | 1. Gently insert a calcium alginate swab into the posterior nasopharynx via the nose. | Direct media inoculation or swab transport | Plates: ≤15 min, RT Swabs: ≤2 h, RT | ≤24 h, RT | 1/day | Inoculated plates should be placed quickly into a $CO_2$ environment. Sinus specimens are collected surgically by needle aspirate, never a swab. Nasopharyngeal and throat specimens do not represent sinus specimen. |

| Specimen | Collection | Transport container | Transport time/temp | No. | Comments |
|---|---|---|---|---|---|
| Throat | 1. Depress the tongue with a tongue depressor. 2. Firmly sample the posterior pharynx, tonsils, and inflamed areas with a sterile swab. | Swab transport | ≤2 h, RT | 1/day | Throat cultures are contraindicated for patients with an inflamed epiglottis. Swabs for *N. gonorrhoeae* should be placed in charcoal-containing transport media and plated ≤12 h after collection. Jembec, Bio-Bags, and a GonoPak are better for transport at RT. |
| Skin: dermatophytosis (51, 69) | 1. Cleanse the affected area with 70% alcohol. 2. Gently scrape the surface of the skin at the active margin (leading edge) of the lesion. *Do not draw blood.* 3. Place the sample in a clean container or between two clean glass slides. | Clean container, enough scrapings to cover the head of a thumbtack | ≤72 h, RT | 1/day/site | If the specimen is submitted between glass slides, tape the slides together and submit in an envelope. Never refrigerate. Dermatophytes are sensitive to cold. |
| Tissue (23) | 1. Submit in a sterile container. 2. For small samples, add several drops of sterile saline to keep moist. *Do not allow tissue to dry out.* 3. Place in an anaerobic transport system or a sterile, moist jar. | Anaerobic transport system or a sterile screw-cap jar. Saline may need to be added. | ≤15 min, RT | None | Always submit as much tissue as possible. If possible, save an amount of surgical tissue at −70°C in case further studies are needed. Never submit a swab that has simply been rubbed over the surface, especially from surgery. For quantitative study, a 2 × 1 cm sample is appropriate, i.e., about 500 mg. Some legionella may be inhibited by saline. |

*(Table continues on next page)*

**Table 18** Bacteriology and mycology specimen collection guidelines[a] *(continued)*

| Specimen type (reference[s]) | Collection | | Time and temp | | Replica limits | Comment(s) |
|---|---|---|---|---|---|---|
| | Guidelines | Device and/or minimum vol | Local transport[b] | Courier or local storage | | |
| Urine | | | | | | More detail for fungal specimen management is found in reference (43). |
| Female, midstream (71) | 1. Thoroughly cleanse the urethral area with soap and water. 2. Rinse the area with wet gauze pads. 3. While holding the labia apart, begin voiding. 4. After several milliliters have passed, collect a midstream portion without stopping the flow of urine. | Sterile wide-mouth container, ≥1 ml, or urine transport kit | Unpreserved: ≤2 h, RT Preserved: ≤24 h, RT | ≤24 h, 4°C | 1/day | Attempts at *Chlamydia* antigen detection in urine from women may be unproductive (72); molecular methods are generally recommended. Urine is toxic to cell lines and, therefore, not the specimen of choice for chlamydiae culture. The midstream portion can be used for bacterial culture. |
| Male, midstream (71) | 1. Cleanse the glans with soap and water. 2. Rinse with wet gauze pads. 3. Holding the foreskin retracted, begin voiding. 4. After several milliliters have passed, collect a midstream portion without stopping the flow of urine. | Sterile wide-mouth container, ≥1 ml, or urine transport kit | Unpreserved: ≤2 h, RT Preserved: ≤24 h, RT | ≤24 h, 4°C | 1/day | The first part of the urine stream is used for probe, antigen, and molecular tests for chlamydiae. Wait 2 h after the last micturition. The midstream portion can be used for culture. |

| | Collection procedure | Container | Transport/storage | | Comments |
|---|---|---|---|---|---|
| Straight catheter (71) | 1. Thoroughly cleanse the urethral area with soap and water. 2. Rinse the area with wet gauze pads. 3. Aseptically, insert a catheter into the bladder. 4. After allowing ~15 ml to pass, collect urine to be submitted in a sterile container. | Sterile, leakproof container | Unpreserved: ≤2 h, RT Preserved: ≤24 h, RT | ≤24 h, 4°C | 1/day | Straight catheters are acceptable specimens but if preparation is inadequate, the procedure may introduce urethral flora into the bladder and increase the risk of iatrogenic infection. |
| Indwelling catheter (71) | 1. Disinfect the catheter collection port with 70% alcohol. 2. Use a needle and syringe to aseptically collect 5–10 ml of urine. 3. Transfer to a sterile tube or container. | Sterile, leakproof container | Unpreserved: ≤2 h, RT Preserved: ≤24 h, RT | ≤24 h, 4°C | 1/day | Foley catheter tips are not acceptable for culture and should not be submitted or accepted. |
| Wound | See Abscess | | | | |

[a]EtOH, ethanol; RT, room temperature; i.v, intravenous; AFB, acid-fast bacilli; CSF, cerebrospinal fluid; BAP, blood agar plate; CHOC, chocolate agar; BHI, brain heart infusion; PVA, poly-vinyl alcohol fixative; TPPA, *Treponema pallidum* particle agglutination; FTA-ABS, fluorescent treponemal antibody-absorbed.

[b]All specimens should be transported in leakproof plastic bags having a separate compartment for the requisition.

**Table 19** Specimen management for infrequently encountered organisms (13, 38, 41, 72)[a]

| Organism(s) | Specimen(s) of choice | Transport issue(s) | Comment(s) |
|---|---|---|---|
| *Afipia* spp. | Blood<br>Tissue<br>Lymph node aspirate | 1 wk, 4°C<br>Indefinitely, −70°C | May see organisms in or on erythrocytes with Giemsa staining. Use Warthin-Starry silver stain for tissue. SPS is toxic. |
| *Bartonella* spp. (cat scratch fever) | Blood: 10 ml in lysis centrifugation tubes | Process within 8 h of collection | Detection of *Bartonella* in blood is extremely difficult even when optimum procedures are used. |
| *Borrelia burgdorferi* (Lyme disease) | Skin biopsy at lesion periphery<br>Serum in clot tube<br>Blood<br>CSF | Keep tissue moist and sterile. Hand-carry to laboratory if possible. | Consider serology in addition to culture, but serology is insensitive for first 14 days of infection. Screen with EIA for IgG and IgM in acute and convalescent sera. Culture yield is low.<br>Use Warthin-Starry silver stain for tissue. Use AO, FA, and Giemsa staining for blood and CSF. |
| *Borrelia* spp. (relapsing fever) | Blood: for thick or thin smears use Wright's or Giemsa stain. Dark-field sometimes helpful with blood.<br>Bone marrow | Transport at RT in EDTA or citrate tube. Process within 30 min if possible.<br>Pediatric lysis-centrifugation tube is helpful. | Routine blood culture bottles are useful if held 30 days. Detection in blood is best when patient is febrile. Can be visualized about 70% of the time. Spirochete load diminishes with each febrile episode.<br>Use joint fluid culture in arthritis.<br>Notify laboratory on suspicion of *Borrelia* spp. |
| *Klebsiella granulomatis* (*Calymmatobacterium* spp.) (granuloma inguinale; donovanosis) | Tissue<br>Subsurface or lesion base scrapings into formalin | Transport at RT. 2 h transport time optimal. | Mostly a tropical disease. Stain with Wright's or Giemsa stain and note blue rods with polar granules. Epithelium alone is inadequate. Culture is nonproductive. |
| *Coxiella* spp. (Q fever), *Rickettsia* spp. (spotted fevers, typhus) | Serum in clot tube for IFA<br>Plasma in EDTA tube for Coxiella NAAT testing.<br>Skin biopsy for NAAT tests<br>Blood | Transport serum/plasma at RT, within 2 h. Blood and tissue should be frozen at −70°C until shipped. Use sterile container on ice for tissue. | Refer isolation to reference laboratory. Serologic diagnosis is preferred. Use IFA for *R. rickettsii* IgM and IgG. |

| Organism | Specimen | Comments |
|---|---|---|
| *Ehrlichia* spp. | Blood smear<br>Skin biopsy<br>Blood (heparin or EDTA)<br>CSF<br>Serum | Serologic diagnosis preferred. Mix smear in methanol. Tissue stained with FA or Gimenez stain. Wright's or Giemsa stain of peripheral blood or buffy coat WBC smear during first week of infection. Refer isolation to reference laboratory. CSF for direct examination and PCR. |
| *Francisella* spp. (tularemia)[b]<br>**Highly infectious and risky to handle specimens** | Lymph node aspirate<br>Scrapings<br>Lesion biopsy<br>Blood<br>Serum – acute and convalescent<br>Sputum | Material for culture should be transported on ice. Keep tissue moist and sterile. Hold at 4°–20°C until tested, or at −70°C for shipment. For PCR test, transport on ice or frozen.<br>Send to reference laboratory or use BSL-3 practices for all manipulations. Serology is helpful. Tissue Gram staining is not productive. IFA is available. Culture is effective 10% of the time. |
| *Leptospira* spp. | Serum<br>Blood (heparin, sodium oxalate, citrate)<br>CSF (first week)<br>Urine (after first week) | Blood <1 h<br>Urine <1 h or dilute 1:10 in 1% bovine serum albumin and storage at 4°–20°C<br>Rapid transport to laboratory or freeze. Ship on dry ice.<br>Collect specimens while patient is febrile. Serology is most helpful. Acidic urine is detrimental. Dark-field and direct FA are useful. Use Warthin-Starry silver stain for tissue. Citrate or EDTA tubes optimum for PCR analysis. Heparin, SPS, and saponin are inhibitory to PCR. |
| *Streptobacillus* spp. (rat bite fever; Haverhill fever) | Blood<br>Aspirates of joint fluid | High-volume bottle preferred<br>Do not refrigerate. Requires blood, serum, or ascetic fluid for growth. SPS is inhibitory. AO stain is helpful. |

[a]SPS, sodium polyanethol sulfonate; AO, acridine orange; FA, fluorescent antibody stain; RT, room temperature; CSF, cerebrospinal fluid; NAAT, nucleic acid amplification test; BSL-3, Biosafety Level 3; IFA, indirect fluorescent antibody stain; WBC, white blood cell.

[b]Laboratory safety hazard.

**Table 20** Specimen guide for virus isolation[a]

| Clinical syndrome | Associated viruses | THR | LES | URN | CSF | FEC | Other specimens | Usefulness of serology | Other agents to consider |
|---|---|---|---|---|---|---|---|---|---|
| Cardiac | Enterovirus[b] | X | | | | X | Heart tissue/fluid | Yes | Enterovirus[b] |
| CNS infection | Enterovirus | X | | | X (NAAT) | X | Rectal swab | No | Arbovirus[c,d] |
| | Parechovirus | | | | X (NAAT) | | | | HIV[c,e] |
| | Herpes simplex 1 and 2 | X | X | | X (NAAT) | | Brain biopsy | No | Measles virus[c] |
| | Mumps virus[b] | X | X | | | | Saliva | Paired sera | Rabies virus[c,e] |
| | Varicella-zoster virus | | X | X | X (NAAT) | | | | Lymphocytic choriomeningitis virus[c] |
| Congenital or neonatal | CMV[b] | X | | X | | | Buffy coat | IgM | Hepatitis B virus[c] |
| | Enterovirus[b] | X | X | X | | X | Rectal swab | No | HIV[c] |
| | Herpes simplex virus[b] | X | X | X | X | | Scraping, DFA | IgM | Parvovirus B19[c] |
| | Varicella-zoster virus[b] | X | X | | X | | | | Rubella virus[c] |
| Gastrointestinal | Adenoviruses[e] 40/41 | | | | | X | Stool/rectal swab | No | Norwalk agents[e] |
| | CMV[b] | | | | | | Biopsy for culture | No | Norovirus |
| | Rotavirus[e] | | | | | X | Stool, rectal swab | No | Sapovirus |
| Genital | Herpes simplex virus[b] | X | X | X | | | Cervix/vulva | No | CMV[b] |
| | Mumps virus[b] (orchitis) | X | | | | | Saliva | Paired sera | Human papillomavirus[e] |
| Mononucleosis | EBV[c] | | | | | | Buffy coat | Yes | Dengue virus[c] |
| Fever of unknown origin | CMV[b] | X | | X | | | Buffy coat | IgM | Hepatitis A–E viruses[c,e] |
| | | | | | | | | | Parvovirus B19 |
| Ocular | Adenovirus[b] | X | | | | | Conjunctival | No | Enterovirus[b] |
| | Herpes simplex virus[b] | X | | | | | Conjunctival | No | CMV[b] |
| | Varicella-zoster virus | | | | | | Corneal swab | Yes | |

Rash

| Syndrome | Virus | | | Specimen | Serology | Other viruses |
|---|---|---|---|---|---|---|
| Maculopapular | Enterovirus[b] | X | | Rectal swab | No | Human herpesvirus 6[c] |
| | Measles/rubeola virus[c] | X | X | Respiratory secretions | Paired sera | Parvovirus B19[c] |
| | | | | | | Rubella virus[c] |
| Vesicular | Enterovirus[b] | X | | | No | |
| | Herpes simplex virus[b,c] | X | | | No | |
| | Varicella-zoster virus[b] | X | | | Paired sera | |
| Respiratory tract infection | Adenovirus[b] | X | | Nasopharynx | No | CMV[b] (in bronchoalveolar lavages) |
| | Enterovirus[b] | X | | Nasopharynx | No | Hantavirus[c] |
| | Influenza virus[b,c] | X | | Nasopharynx | No | |
| | Parainfluenza virus[b] | X | | Nasopharynx | No | |
| | Respiratory syncytial virus[e] | X | | Nasopharynx | No | |
| | Rhinovirus[b] | X | | Nasopharynx | No | |

[a] CNS, central nervous system; HIV, human immunodeficiency virus; CMV, cytomegalovirus; DFA, direct fluorescent antibody; EBV, Epstein-Barr virus; THR, throat; LES, lesion; URN, urine; CSF, cerebrospinal fluid; FEC, feces.

[b] Virus isolation: method of choice for diagnosis. "Enterovirus" includes the historical designation of echovirus and coxsackie A and B viruses.

[c] Serology: method of choice for diagnosis.

[d] Includes western equine, eastern equine, St. Louis, and California encephalitis viruses.

[e] Antigen/nucleic acid detection methods available.

**Table 21** Virology specimen collection guidelines[a]

| Specimen type (references) | Collection | | Transport time and temperature | Replica limits | Comment(s) |
|---|---|---|---|---|---|
| | Guidelines | Device and minimum volume | | | |
| For virus specimen selection guidelines, refer to Table 7 (14, 23, 73, 74) | In general, specimens for virus detection should be collected within 4 days after onset of illness, because virus shedding decreases rapidly after that time. With only a *rare* exception, virus cultures are not worthwhile for specimens collected more than 7 days after the onset of illness. | Except for body fluids (BAL, CSF, urine, blood), place all viral specimens in VTM. | Most viruses remain stable at 4°C for 2–3 days, and almost indefinitely at –70°C. *Do not freeze specimens at –20°C.* | | To ensure proper evaluation, always require the following information: (i) date of illness onset, (ii) date and time specimen was collected, (iii) admitting diagnosis. Collection of acute- and convalescent-phase sera should always be considered. |
| Blood (14, 73) | 1. Cleanse venipuncture site with 70% isopropyl alcohol. Follow instructions for using chlorhexidine preparation or continue as below: 2. Starting at the site, swab concentrically with 2% iodine tincture. 3. Allow the iodine to dry (~1 min). 4. *Do not palpate the vein at this point.* 5. Collect 8–10 ml in an anticoagulant tube (viral transport is *not* required). 6. After venipuncture, remove iodine from the skin with alcohol. | Citrate, EDTA, or heparin tube, 8–10 ml/tube. You may need to draw ≥2 tubes from patients who are leukopenic. | Submit at RT | None | Frequently identified: CMV, HSV Less frequently identified: arboviruses, arenaviruses, EBV, HIV-1, enterovirus (newborn), Zika virus Collect blood during the early, acute phase of infection. For specimens requiring cell separation, maintain at RT. *Do not refrigerate.* Always refer to and follow CDC or state public health recommendations for specimen management of emerging pathogens such as Zika and Ebola virus. |

| Specimen | Procedure | Transport | Quantity | Comments |
|---|---|---|---|---|
| CSF (23, 58, 75) | 1. Disinfect site with 2% iodine tincture.<br>2. Insert a needle with stylet at L3-L4, L4-L5, or L5-S1 interspace.<br>3. On reaching the subarachnoid space, remove the stylet and collect 2–5 ml in a sterile leakproof tube (VTM not required). | Sterile screw-cap tube, 1.0 ml | Submit immediately at 4°C. | None | Frequently identified: coxsackievirus (some), echovirus, enterovirus, mumps virus<br>Less frequently identified: arboviruses, HSV, LCMV, rabies virus |
| Cervical or vaginal swab[b] (14, 23, 73) | 1. If lesions are present, swab vigorously. Place swab in VTM.<br>2. If lesions are not present, remove mucus from the cervix with a swab and discard the swab.<br>3. Firmly sample the endocervix (~1 cm into the cervical canal) with a fresh swab by rotating the swab for 5 s.<br>4. Place swab in VTM.<br>5. Perform a vulvar sweep using a second swab; place both swabs in the same transport tube. | Swab[b] | Immediately place swab in VTM. Submit at 4°C. | 1/day/source | Frequently identified: HSV, CMV<br>Noncultivable: papillomavirus, molluscum contagiosum virus<br>Although a cervical swab sample is the specimen of choice in the monitoring of pregnant women with a history of genital HSV infection, recovery of HSV may be increased by also sampling the vulva. |
| Conjunctiva swab[b] (14, 23, 73) | 1. Collect material from the lower conjunctiva with a flexible, fine-shafted swab moistened with sterile saline.<br>2. Place swab in VTM. | Swab[b] | Immediately place swab in VTM. Submit at 4°C. | None | Frequently identified: adenovirus; coxsackievirus A (some), CMV, HSV, enterovirus (including type 70), Newcastle disease virus<br>Only a small amount of specimen will be retrieved by a swab of the conjunctiva. |

*(Table continues on next page)*

**Table 21** Virology specimen collection guidelines[a] (*continued*)

| Specimen type (references) | Collection | | Transport time and temperature | Replica limits | Comment(s) |
|---|---|---|---|---|---|
| | Guidelines | Device and minimum volume | | | |
| Feces (23, 76, 77) | 1. Pass directly into a clean, dry container.<br>2. Add sufficient VTM to prevent drying, or transfer 2–4 g of stool to sterile, leakproof container and transport immediately to laboratory. | Sterile, leakproof, wide-mouth container; ≥2 g | Transfer to 8–10 ml VTM.<br>Submit at 4°C. | 1/day | Frequently identified: adenoviruses; enteroviruses<br>Less frequently isolated: rotavirus<br>Rotavirus antigen is detected by EIA. |
| Nasal swab[b] (14, 23, 73) | 1. Pass a flexible, fine-shafted swab 1–2 cm into the nostril. A flocked swab may be best.<br>2. Rotate slowly for 5 s to absorb secretions.<br>3. Remove swab and place in VTM.<br>4. Repeat for other nostril using a fresh swab. Place both swabs in the same transport tube. | Swab[b] | Immediately place swab in VTM.<br>Submit at 4°C. | 1/day | Frequently identified: influenza virus, parainfluenza virus, rhinovirus (limited), RSV (nasopharyngeal preferred)<br>Influenza A virus and RSV are usually detected by molecular methods or antigen detection.<br>For influenza testing, nasal and nasopharyngeal washes may be more effective unless a flocked swab is used. |
| Nasopharynx aspirate or wash (14, 23, 73) | 1. Pass appropriate size tubing or catheter into the nasopharynx.<br>2. Aspirate material with a small syringe.<br>3. If material cannot be aspirated, tilt patient's head back about 70° and instill 3–7 ml of sterile saline or VTM until it occludes the nostril.<br>4. Reaspirate. If <2 ml, deposit aspirate in VTM. If >2 ml, no VTM is required.<br>5. Place specimen at 4°C immediately. | Viral transport tube | Immediately place 8–10 ml in VTM.<br>Submit at 4°C. | 1/day | Frequently identified: influenza virus, parainfluenza virus, rhinovirus (limited), RSV<br>Influenza A virus and RSV are usually detected by molecular methods or antigen detection.<br>Turnaround time for influenza virus shell-vial culture is 24–48 h. |

| Specimen | Collection procedure | Swab | Storage | Frequency | Viruses |
|---|---|---|---|---|---|
| Nasopharynx swab[b] (14, 23, 73) | Estimate the distance to the nasopharynx as about half the distance from the base of the nose to the ear. 1. Pass a flexible, fine-shafted swab into the nasopharynx until resistance is felt. 2. Allow secretions to absorb for 5 s; then carefully remove swab and place it in VTM. 3. Repeat for other nostril using a fresh swab. Place both swabs in the same transport tube. | Swab[b] | Immediately place swab in VTM. Submit at 4°C. | 1/day | Frequently identified: influenza virus, parainfluenza virus, rhinovirus (limited), RSV. Patients, especially children, may be uncomfortable during the procedure so be prepared and be quick, but the specimen must represent the nasopharynx, not the back of the nares. |
| Oral swab[b] | 1. Firmly sample base of an oral lesion(s) with a swab. 2. Place swab in VTM. | Swab[b] | Immediately place swab in VTM. Submit at 4°C. | 1/day | Frequently identified: enterovirus (some), HSV |
| Rash | | | | | |
| Maculopapular (14, 23, 73) | 1. Gently cleanse area with sterile saline. 2. Disrupt the surface of the lesion and firmly sample its base with a swab moistened with sterile saline. 3. Place swab in VTM. | Swab[b] | Immediately place swab in VTM. Submit at 4°C. | 1/day/source | Frequently identified: adenovirus, enterovirus, rubella virus, measles virus (rubeola virus). Less frequently identified: poxviruses. Noncultivable: parvovirus B19 |
| Vesicular (14, 23, 73) | 1. Sample only *fresh* vesicles because older crusted vesicles may not contain viable virus. 2. Cleanse area with sterile saline. 3. Carefully open the vesicle with needle or scalpel blade. 4. Using a swab, collect fluid and cellular material by vigorously sampling the base of the lesion. 5. Place in VTM. | Swab[b] | Immediately place swab in VTM. Submit at 4°C. | 1/day/source | Frequently identified: enterovirus (some), echovirus, HSV, VZV. Less frequently identified: poxviruses. The preferred specimen for VZV is a vesicle aspirate placed in 1 ml VTM. |

*(Table continues on next page)*

**Table 21** Virology specimen collection guidelines[a] (continued)

| Specimen type (references) | Collection | | Transport time and temperature | Replica limits | Comment(s) |
|---|---|---|---|---|---|
| | Guidelines | Device and minimum volume | | | |
| Throat swab[b] | 1. Using a tongue depressor, depress the tongue to prevent contamination with saliva, cheeks, or gums.<br>2. Firmly sample the posterior pharynx, tonsils, and inflamed areas with a sterile swab.<br>3. Place swab in VTM. | Swab[b] | Immediately place swab in VTM. Submit at 4°C. | 1/day | Frequently identified: adenovirus, CMV, enterovirus, HSV, influenza A and B viruses, measles virus, mumps virus, parainfluenza virus<br>Less frequently identified: RSV |
| Tissue (14, 23, 73) | 1. Obtain tissue/biopsy samples from areas directly adjacent to affected tissue.<br>2. Place specimen in a sterile vial containing VTM. | VTM | Submit at 4°C. | None | Always submit as much tissue as possible. *Never* submit a swab that has simply been rubbed over the surface. |
| Urethral swab[b] | Patient should not have urinated ≤1 h prior to collection.<br>1. Express and discard any exudate.<br>2. Carefully insert flexible, fine-shafted swab 4 cm into urethra.<br>3. Rotate swab 2–3 times to obtain an adequate number of cells.<br>4. Remove swab and place in VTM. | Swab[b] | Immediately place swab in VTM. Submit at 4°C. | 1/day | Frequently identified: CMV, HSV<br>Exudate from male urethra (but not female) may be Gram stained for additional recognition of possible *Neisseria gonorrhoeae*. The exudate is not tested for viral etiology. |

| Specimen | Collection | Container | Transport | Frequency | Viruses |
|---|---|---|---|---|---|
| Urine | Refer to the guidelines for urine collection. Collect at least 5 ml of midstream clean, voided urine in a sterile container (VTM not required). | Sterile container, 5 ml | Submit at 4°C. | 1/day | Frequently identified: adenovirus, CMV, HSV, mumps virus Less frequently identified: polyomavirus (JC virus), rubella virus Molecular methods are usually performed for detection of CMV from urine, however, if viral culture is used, two or three specimens on successive days can maximize recovery of CMV. |

---

[a]BAL, bronchoalveolar lavage; CSF, cerebral spinal fluid; VTM, viral transport medium; RT, room temperature; CMV, cytomegalovirus; HSV, herpes simplex virus; EBV, Epstein-Barr virus; HIV-1, human immunodeficiency virus type 1; LCMV, lymphocytic choriomeningitis virus; EIA, enzyme immunoassay; RSV, respiratory syncytial virus; ELISA, enzyme-linked immunosorbent assay; VZV, varicella-zoster virus.

[b]Dacron-, rayon-, or cotton-tipped swabs with plastic or aluminum shafts are acceptable; calcium alginate swabs or swabs with wooden shafts are not acceptable.

**Table 22** Parasitology: anatomic sites containing diagnostic stages

| Parasite | Site of diagnostic stage[a] | | | | | | | | | |
|---|---|---|---|---|---|---|---|---|---|---|
| | BLD | CNS | Eye | GI | L/S | Lung | LN | MUS | Skin | Other |
| *Acanthamoeba* spp. | | X | X | | | | | | X (rare) | |
| *Ascaris* larvae | | | | | | X | | | | |
| *Balamuthia mandrillaris* | | X | | | | | | | X | |
| *Babesia* spp. | RBS | | | | | | | | | |
| *Cyclospora* spp. | | | | X | | | | | | |
| *Cryptosporidium parvum* | | | | X | X | | | | | |
| *Echinococcus* spp. | | X | | | X | X | | | | |
| *Entamoeba histolytica* | | | | X | X | | | | | |
| *Fasciola hepatica* | | | | X | X | | | | | Bile duct |
| *Hartmannella* spp. | | X | | | | | | | | |
| Hookworm, larvae | | | | | | X | | | | |
| *Leishmania donovani* | WBC | | | | X | | X | | | Bone marrow |
| *Leishmania* spp.[b] | | | | | | | | | X | |
| *Loa loa* | | | X | | | | | | | Calabar swellings |
| Microfilariae | Plasma | | | | | | X[c] | | X[d] | |
| Microsporidia | | | X | X | | X | | X | | Urogenital |

| Organism | Specimen | BLD | CNS | GI | L/S | LN | MUS | Skin | Other |
|---|---|---|---|---|---|---|---|---|---|
| *Naegleria* spp. | | | X[e] | | | | | | |
| *Onchocerca volvulus* | | | | | | | | X[d] | |
| *Opisthorchis sinensis*[f] | | | | X | X | | | | |
| *Paragonimus westermani* | | | | X | | | | | |
| *Plasmodium* spp. | RBC | X | | | | | | | |
| *Schistosoma* spp. | | | | X | | | | | Urogenital |
| *Strongyloides* larvae | | | | X | | | | | |
| *Taenia solium* | | | X[g] | X[g] | | | | | |
| *Toxoplasma gondii* | WBC | X | X | | | X | | | |
| *Trichinella spiralis* | | | | | | | X | | |
| *Trichomonas vaginalis* | | | | | | | | | Urogenital |
| *Trypanosoma cruzi* | Plasma | X | | | | | | | Heart |
| *Trypanosoma* spp.[h] | Plasma | X | X | | | | | | |

[a]BLD, blood; CNS, central nervous system; GI, gastrointestinal; L/S, liver/spleen; LN, lymph node; MUS, muscle; RBC, red blood cell; WBC, white blood cell.

[b]Includes *L. tropica*, *L. Mexicana* complex, and *L. braziliensis* complex.

[c]*Wuchereria bancrofti* and *Brugia malayi*.

[d]Skin snips for *M. streptocerca* and *O. volvulus*.

[e]*Naegleria fowleri*.

[f]*Clonorchis sinensis*.

[g]Cysticerci.

[h]Includes *Trypanosoma brucei gambiense* and *T. brucei rhodesiense*.

**Table 23** Parasitology specimen collection guidelines (23, 28, 78–80)

| Specimen type (references) | Collection[a] | | | | Replica limits | Transport time and temp | Comments |
|---|---|---|---|---|---|---|---|
| | Guidelines | Device | Preservative | Minimum vol | | | |
| **Blood** Direct smear | 1. Warm the patient's hands by covering them with a hot moist towel, by immersing them in warm water, or by rubbing them together briskly. 2. Disinfect the palmar surface of the tip of the middle or "ring" finger with gauze soaked with 70% alcohol (do not use cotton because it may introduce artifacts). 3. Allow alcohol to *dry completely*, because residual alcohol does not permit a drop of blood to "round up" and may also fix the red blood cells, rendering the thick smear unsuitable for staining. 4. Puncture the palmar area with a sterile disposable lancet, resulting in free-flowing blood. | *Wear gloves when preparing thin or thick films.* Thin-smear preparation: 1. Place one drop of blood near one end of a slide. 2. Hold another slide at a 45° angle and draw it into the drop of blood. 3. Allow the blood to spread the width of the slide and then rapidly push the spreader slide to the opposite end, producing a feathered smear. 4. Label slide, dry at RT, and stain as soon as visibly dry. Thick-smear preparation: 1. Touch a slide to a drop of blood (rounded up on the finger). 2. Rotate the slide to form a circular film about the size of a nickel. (For blood without anticoagulant, stir blood 20–30 s to prevent formation of a fibrin clot.) | | | | Malaria: STAT Other: ≤2 h, RT | Optimal time to obtain smear *Babesia* spp.: any time *Brugia malayi*[b]: ~midnight *Leishmania donovani*[b]: any time *Loa loa*[b]: ~noon *Mansonella ozzardi*[b]: day or night *Mansonella perstans*[b]: night better than day *Plasmodium* spp.[c]: between chills *Trypanosoma cruzi*[b]: acute stage *Trypanosoma brucei gambiense*[b,d]: acute stage *Trypanosoma brucei rhodesiense*[b,d]: acute stage *Wuchereria bancrofti*[b]: ~midnight; additional smears obtained 6, 12, or 24 h after admission may be necessary. |
| Venipuncture | 1. For buffy coat concentration of filariasis, trypanosomiasis, and, to a lesser extent, leishmaniasis, collect 10 ml of whole blood with heparin or EDTA (0.002 g/10 ml of blood). 2. Submit directly (≤15 min) to the laboratory at RT. 3. Thick or thin smears should be obtained via finger puncture; see above. | Vacutainer | Heparin: filariasis, *Trypanosoma* spp. EDTA: malaria; see Comments | ≥10 ml | 1/day | ≤15 min, RT | Common parasites: *L. donovani*, *Trypanosoma* spp., microfilariae Venipuncture for malaria is common but *not* recommended because smears must be made within 1 h to detect stippling. However, this approach is common, and personnel learn to identify with or without stippling. |

| Specimen | Collection | Container | | Volume | | Transport | Common parasites |
|---|---|---|---|---|---|---|---|
| CSF, CNS | See "Specimen type: CSF" (Table 15) for specific guidelines for obtaining a CSF specimen. | Sterile tube | None | ≥1 ml | None | ≤15 min, RT | Common parasites: *Acanthamoeba* spp., *Balamuthia mandrillaris*, *Echinococcus* spp., larval cestodes, microsporidia, *Naegleria fowleri*, *Taenia solium*, *Toxoplasma gondii*, *Trypanosoma* spp. |
| Duodenal aspirate | 1. Obtain a specimen via nasogastric intubation or with a string test (Entero-Test capsule). 2. Place aspirate in a sterile centrifuge tube and transport it directly (≤15 min) to the laboratory since specimens must be examined within 1 h of collection. | Sterile centrifuge tube | None | ≥2 ml | None | ≤15 min, RT | Common parasites: *Clonorchis sinensis* (eggs), *Cryptosporidium parvum* (oocyst), *Giardia lamblia* (trophozoite), *Isospora belli* (oocyst), *Strongyloides* spp. (larvae) For the string test, the patient swallows a gelatin capsule attached to a long string. The end of the string remains outside the mouth and is taped to the cheek. The capsule dissolves in the stomach and the string passes into the upper part of the small intestine (duodenum). The string is left in place for 4–6 h or overnight. Then it is withdrawn and the end is examined under the microscope for parasites that are attached to it. |

*(Table continues on next page)*

**Table 23** Parasitology specimen collection guidelines (23, 28, 78–80) (*continued*)

| Specimen type (references) | Collection^a | | Preservative | Minimum vol | Replica limits | Transport time and temp | Comments |
|---|---|---|---|---|---|---|---|
| | Guidelines | Device | | | | | |
| Eye: corneal scraping for *Acanthamoeba* spp. (38, 61) | 1. Instill two drops of local anesthetic into the conjunctival sac and/or onto the corneal epithelium. 2. Using a sterile spatula, scrape ulcers or lesions and either inoculate a nonnutrient agar plate directly or place scraping in Page's saline and transport to the laboratory. 3. Apply remaining material to two clean glass slides for staining and fix immediately with 95% ethanol (cysts may become airborne when allowed to air-dry). | Direct inoculation of nonnutrient agar coated with bacterial overlay or Page's ameba saline. | Page's ameba saline | None | None | ≤15 min, RT | Common parasites: *Acanthamoeba* spp., *Naegleria* spp. If necessary, contact lenses, lens cases, and all opened solutions may be evaluated for *Acanthamoeba* by stains (28). |
| Feces | | | | | | | |
| Preserved (39, 81) | 1. Pass directly into a clean, dry container. 2. Specimens that cannot be examined within the recommended time must be transferred to an appropriate preservative (FOR, MIF, SAF, PVA). Mix well and allow to stand at RT for 30 min for adequate fixation. 3. For unpreserved specimens, the transport times must correspond to the recommendations provided below. 4. Submit three specimens over 7–10 days because shedding may be intermittent. | Sterile, leakproof, wide-mouth container | FOR + PVA or MIF + PVA or SAF or other one-vial system Hold at RT for 30 min for fixation. | 1 part feces to 3 parts fixative | 1/day | Indefinite, RT | Common parasites: helminths, protozoa Unacceptable stool specimen: (i) Contaminated with urine or water (e.g., from diapers); (ii) nonpuncturable or dried specimen; (iii) specimens containing bismuth, barium, magnesia, mineral oil, or gallbladder dye |

| | | | | | | | |
|---|---|---|---|---|---|---|---|
| Unpreserved (39, 81) | Parasite and cyclical peak: *Ascaris lumbricoides*, constant *Dientamoeba fragilis*, irregular *Diphyllobothrium latum*, irregular *E. histolytica*, 7–10 days *Giardia lamblia*, 3–7 days Hookworm, constant *Trichuris trichiura*, constant *Schistosoma* spp., irregular | Sterile, leakproof, wide-mouth container | None[a] | 5 g | 1/day | Liquid: ≤30 min, RT Semisolid: ≤1 h, RT Formed: ≤24 h, 4°C | The general waiting period necessary to allow substances to clear is 7 days, except for gallbladder dye which may require 21 days. |
| Pinworm paddle (81) | 1. Gently press the paddle's sticky side against several areas of the perianal region while spreading open the perianal folds. 2. Place the paddle in the transport container and tighten the cap. 3. Daily consecutive specimens (≥6) should be obtained before patient is considered infection free. | Pinworm paddle kit | None | None | 1/day | ≤24 h, RT | Common parasites: *Enterobius vermicularis, Taenia* spp. Specimens are best obtained at 10–11 p.m. or upon waking and before a bowel movement or bath. Wash hands after collection. |
| Skin snip (13) | 1. A sharp razor blade can be used to obtain a sample of skin which may be so superficial that no bleeding occurs. 2. Alternatively, a needle can be used to raise the skin and with a scalpel remove the skin below the needle. 3. Any body location is satisfactory, but the middorsal region just to one side of midline is frequently selected. 4. Place the skin snip in a tube containing 0.2–0.4 ml of saline. | Sterile tube | Sterile saline | None | None | ≤15 min, RT | Common parasites: *Mansonella streptocerca, Onchocerca volvulus* |

(Table continues on next page)

**Table 23** Parasitology specimen collection guidelines (23, 28, 78–80) *(continued)*

| Specimen type (references) | Collection[a] | | | Minimum vol | Replica limits | Transport time and temp | Comments |
|---|---|---|---|---|---|---|---|
| | Guidelines | Device | Preservative | | | | |
| Skin ulcer | 1. Obtain scrapings or biopsies of the active margin of cutaneous or mucocutaneous ulcers. A punch biopsy is recommended.<br>2. Place sample in a sterile tube containing enough sterile saline to keep it moist. | Sterile tube | Sterile saline | None | 1/day/site | ≤15 min, RT | Common parasites: *Acanthamoeba* spp.; *Entamoeba histolytica*; *Leishmania* spp. If cultures will be used for *Leishmania* spp., specimen must not be contaminated with bacteria |
| Urine<br>*Schistosoma* spp. | Peak egg excretion occurs between noon and 3 p.m.<br>1. Collect a midday urine specimen in a sterile container.<br>2. In patients with hematuria, eggs are associated with the terminal (last-voided) portion of the specimen containing mucus and blood. | Sterile leakproof container | None | Entire midday urine | 1/day | ≤2 h, RT | Parasites: *Schistosoma haematobium*; *Strongyloides stercoralis*; *Trichomonas vaginalis*; *Wuchereria bancrofti* |

| Organism | Procedure | Container | Preservative | Amount | Frequency | Transport time and temperature | Comments |
|---|---|---|---|---|---|---|---|
| *Trichomonas* | Trophozoites can be found in the urine of both males and females. 1. For males, prostatic massage may be useful. 2. Collect first-voided urine in a sterile container. 3. Transport it to the laboratory <1 h at RT. If transportation will be delayed, centrifuge at 500 × g for 5 min, remove supernatant, overlay sediment with 0.2 ml of sterile saline, and transport at RT. 4. The sediment can also be smeared on a microscope slide, air dried, and stained (Papanicolaou). | Sterile, leakproof container | None | Entire void | 1/day | ≤1 h, RT Do not refrigerate | Specimens must be held at RT and processed within 1 h of collection. Alternatively, the centrifuged pellet may be adsorbed onto a Dacron swab and transported in Amies medium, in which the organisms remain viable for ~24 h. *Do not use calcium alginate swabs.* Commercial "pouch" methods are available for relatively easy transport and culture. Papanicolaou smears may be difficult to interpret for *Trichomonas* spp. |

[a]RT, room temperature; CSF, cerebrospinal fluid; CNS, central nervous system; FOR, 10% formalin; MIF, merthiolate-iodine-formalin; SAF, sodium acetate-formalin; PVA, polyvinyl alcohol.

[b]Collect 10 ml of heparinized blood for buffy coat concentration.

[c]Additional smears obtained 6, 12, or 24 h after admission may be necessary.

[d]CSF is specimen of choice for patients infected >6 months.

# References

1. **Bartlett RC.** 1985. Quality control, p 14–23. *In* Lennette EH, et al (ed), *Manual of Clinical Microbiology*, 4th ed. American Society for Microbiology, Washington, DC.

2. **Carson JA.** 2016. Wound cultures, Procedure 3.13. *In* Leber A (ed), *Clinical Microbiology Procedures Handbook*, 4th ed. ASM Press, Washington, DC.

3. **Lipsky BA, Berendt AR, Deery HG, Embil JM, Joseph WS, Karchmer AW, LeFrock JL, Lew DP, Mader JT, Norden C, Tan JS, Infectious Diseases Society of America.** 2004. Diagnosis and treatment of diabetic foot infections. *Clin Infect Dis* **39**:885–910.

4. **Lawrence JC, Ameen H.** 1998. Swabs and other sampling techniques. *J Wound Care* **7**:232–233.

5. **Perry JL, Ballou DR, Salyer JL.** 1997. Inhibitory properties of a swab transport device. *J Clin Microbiol* **35**:3367–3368.

6. **Helstad AG, Kimball JL, Maki DG.** 1977. Recovery of anaerobic, facultative, and aerobic bacteria from clinical specimens in three anaerobic transport systems. *J Clin Microbiol* **5**:564–569.

7. **Basak S, Dutta SK, Gupta S, Ganguly AC, De R.** 1992. Bacteriology of wound infection: evaluation by surface swab and quantitative full thickness wound biopsy culture. *J Indian Med Assoc* **90**:33–34.

8. **Veen MR, Bloem RM, Petit PL.** 1994. Sensitivity and negative predictive value of swab cultures in musculoskeletal allograft procurement. *Clin Orthop Relat Res* (300):259–263.

9. **Gardner SE, Frantz RA, Saltzman CL, Hillis SL, Park H, Scherubel M.** 2006. Diagnostic validity of three swab techniques for identifying chronic wound infection. *Wound Repair Regen* **14**:548–557.

10. **Parikh AR, Hamilton S, Sivarajan V, Withey S, Butler PE.** 2007. Diagnostic fine-needle aspiration in postoperative wound infections is more accurate at predicting causative organisms than wound swabs. *Ann R Coll Surg Engl* **89**:166–167.

11. **Sapico FL, Canawati HN, Witte JL, Montgomerie JZ, Wagner FW Jr, Bessman AN.** 1980. Quantitative aerobic and anaerobic bacteriology of infected diabetic feet. *J Clin Microbiol* **12**:413–420.

12. **Miller JM, Astles R, Baszler T, Chapin K, Carey R, Garcia L, Gray L, Larone D, Pentella M, Pollock A, Shapiro DS, Weirich E, Wiedbrauk D; Biosafety Blue Ribbon Panel; Centers for Disease Control and Prevention (CDC).** 2012. Guidelines for safe work practices in human and animal medical diagnostic laboratories. Recommendations of a CDC-convened, biosafety blue ribbon panel. MMWR Suppl **61:**1–102.

13. **Leber A (ed).** 2016. *Clinical Microbiology Procedures Handbook*, 4th ed, vol 1 and 2. American Society for Microbiology, Washington, DC.

14. **Johnson FB.** 1990. Transport of viral specimens. *Clin Microbiol Rev* **3:**120–131.

15. **Holden J, Hall GS.** 2007. Collection and transport of clinical specimens for anaerobic culture. *In* Garcia LS (ed), *Clinical Microbiology Procedures Handbook.* American Society for Microbiology, Washington, DC.

16. **Miller JM.** 1999. *A Guide to Specimen Management in Clinical Microbiology*, 2nd ed. American Society for Microbiology, Washington, DC.

17. **Clinical and Laboratory Standards Institute.** 2012. *GP17-A3. Clinical Laboratory Safety; Approved Guideline; Third informational supplement.* Clinical and Laboratory Standards Institute, Villanova, PA.

18. **Clinical and Laboratory Standards Institute.** 2014. *M29-A4. Protection of Laboratory Workers From Occupationally Acquired Infections; Approved Guideline; Fourth informational supplement.* Clinical and Laboratory Standards Institute, Villanova, PA.

19. **Clinical and Laboratory Standards Institute.** 2015. *M100-S25. Performance standards for antimicrobial susceptibility testing; Twenty-fifth informational supplement.* Clinical and Laboratory Standards Institute, Villanova, PA.

20. **Hagen JC, Wood WS, Hashimoto T.** 1977. Effect of temperature on survival of *Bacteroides fragilis* subsp. *fragilis* and *Escherichia coli* in pus. *J Clin Microbiol* **6:**567–570.

21. **Humphries RM, Linscott AJ.** 2015. Laboratory diagnosis of bacterial gastroenteritis. *Clin Microbiol Rev* **28:**3–31.

22. **Lew F, LeBaron CW, Glass RG, Torok T, Griffin PM, Wells JG, Juranek DD, Wahlquist SP.** 1990. Recommendations for the collection of laboratory specimens associated with outbreaks of gastroenteritis. *MMWR* **39**(RR-14)**:**1–13.

23. **Baron EJ, Miller JM, Weinstein MP, Richter SS, Gilligan PH, Thomson RB Jr, Bourbeau P, Carroll KC, Kehl SC, Dunne WM, Robinson-Dunn B, Schwartzman JD, Chapin KC, Snyder JW, Forbes BA, Patel R, Rosenblatt JE, Pritt BS.** 2013. A guide to utilization of the microbiology laboratory for diagnosis of infectious diseases: 2013 recommendations by the Infectious Diseases Society of America (IDSA) and the American Society for Microbiology (ASM)(a). *Clin Infect Dis* **57:**e22–e121.

24. **Morris AJ, Tanner DC, Reller LB.** 1993. Rejection criteria for endotracheal aspirates from adults. *J Clin Microbiol* **31:**1027–1029.

25. **Matkoski C, Sharp SE, Kiska DL.** 2006. Evaluation of the Q score and Q234 systems for cost-effective and clinically relevant interpretation of wound cultures. *J Clin Microbiol* **44:**1869–1872.

26. **Baron EJ, Cassell GH, Duffy LB, Eschembach DA, Greenwood JR, Harvey SM, Madinger NE, Peterson EM, Waites KB.** 1993. Cumitech 17A. Laboratory Diagnosis of Female Genital Tract Infections. *Coordinating ed*, Baron EJ. American Society for Microbiology, Washington, DC.

27. **Baron EJ, Weinstein MP, Dunne WM Jr, Yagupsky P, Welch DF, Wilson DM.** 2005. Cumitech 1C. Blood Cultures IV. *Coordinating ed*, Baron EJ. American Society for Microbiology, Washington, DC.

28. **Garcia LS.** 2007. *Diagnostic Medical Parasitology*, 5th ed. American Society for Microbiology, Washington, DC.

29. **Miller JM, Graves RK.** 1984. Predictive value of culturing gastric aspirates of newborns and placental membranes. *Clin Microbiol Newsl* **6:**125–126.

30. **Nugent RP, Krohn MA, Hillier SL.** 1991. Reliability of diagnosing bacterial vaginosis is improved by a standardized method of gram stain interpretation. *J Clin Microbiol* **29:**297–301.

31. **Meares EM, Stamey TA.** 1968. Bacteriologic localization patterns in bacterial prostatitis and urethritis. *Invest Urol* **5:**492.

32. **Nickel JC, Shoskes D, Wang Y, Alexander RB, Fowler JE Jr, Zeitlin S, O'Leary MP, Pontari MA, Schaeffer AJ, Landis JR, Nyberg L, Kusek JW, Propert KJ.** 2006. How does the pre-massage and post-massage 2-glass test compare to the Meares-Stamey 4-glass test in men with chronic prostatitis/chronic pelvic pain syndrome? *J Urol* **176:**119–124.

33. **Chapman AS, Bakken JS, Folk SM, Paddock CD, Bloch KC, Krusell A, Sexton DJ, Buckingham SC, Marshall GS, Storch GA, Dasch GA, McQuiston JH, Swerdlow DL, Dumler SJ, Nicholson WL, Walker DH, Eremeeva ME, Ohl CA, Tickborne Rickettsial Diseases Working Group, CDC.** 2006. Diagnosis and management of tickborne rickettsial diseases: Rocky Mountain spotted fever, ehrlichioses, and anaplasmosis—United States: a practical guide for physicians and other health-care and public health professionals. *MMWR Recomm Rep* **55**(RR-4):1–27.

34. **Forman MS, Valsamakis A.** 2011. Specimen collection, transport, and processing: virology, p 1276–1288. *In* Versalovic J, Carroll KC, Funke G, Jorgensen JH, Landry ML, Warnock DW (ed), *Manual of Clinical Microbiology*, 10th ed. American Society for Microbiology, Washington, DC.

35. **Wilson ML.** 1996. General principles of specimen collection and transport. *CID* **22:**766–777.

36. **Hambling MH.** 1964. Survival of the respiratory syncytial virus during storage under various conditions. *Br J Exp Pathol* **45:**647–655.

37. **Romanowski EG, Bartels SP, Vogel R, Wetherall NT, Hodges-Savola C, Kowalski RP, Yates KA, Kinchington PR, Gordon YJ.** 2004. Feasibility of an antiviral clinical trial requiring cross-country shipment of conjunctival adenovirus cultures and recovery of infectious virus. *Curr Eye Res* **29:**195–199.

38. **Gray LD, Gilligan PH, Fowler WC.** 2011. Cumitech 13B. Laboratory Diagnosis of Ocular Infections. *Coordinating ed*, Snyder JW. American Society for Microbiology, Washington, DC.

39. **Melvin DM, Brooke MM.** 1982. *Laboratory Procedures for the Diagnosis of Intestinal Parasites*, 3rd ed. HHS publication no. (CDC) 82-8282. US Department of Health and Human Services, Atlanta, GA.

40. **Ellner PD.** 1978. *Current Procedures in Clinical Bacteriology*. Charles C Thomas, Springfield, IL.

41. **Forbes BA, Sahm DF, Weisfeld AS.** 2007. In *Bailey & Scott's Diagnostic Microbiology*, 12th ed, p 784–786. Mosby Elsevier, St. Louis, MO.

42. **McHardy IH, Wu M, Shimizu-Cohen R, Couturier MR, Humphries RM.** 2014. Detection of intestinal protozoa in the clinical laboratory. *J Clin Microbiol* **52:**712–720.

43. **McGowan KL.** 2011. Specimen collection, transport, and processing: mycology, p 1756–1766. *In* Versalovic J, Carroll KC, Funke G, Jorgensen JH, Landry ML, Warnock DW (ed), *Manual of Clinical Microbiology*, 10th ed. American Society for Microbiology, Washington, DC.

44. **Edwards MS.** 1992. Infections due to human and animal bites, p 2234–2345. *In* Feigin RD, Cherry JD (ed), *Textbook of Pediatric Infectious Diseases*, 3rd ed. The W B Saunders Co, Philadelphia.

45. **Goldstein EJC.** 1989. Bite infections, p 455–463. *In* Finegold SW, George WL (ed), *Anaerobic Infections in Humans*. Academic Press, Inc, San Diego, CA.

46. **Ellis CJ.** 1991. The use and abuse of blood cultures. *Infect Dis Newsl* **10:**27–30.

47. **Kirn TJ, Weinstein MP.** 2013. Update on blood cultures: how to obtain, process, report, and interpret. *Clin Microbiol Infect* **19:**513–520.

48. **Riley JA, Weinstein MP.** 1991. Laboratory diagnosis of bacteremia and endocarditis. *Infect Dis Newsl* **10:**4–6.

49. **Ryan MR, Murray PR.** 1993. Historical evolution of automated blood culture systems. *Clin Microbiol Newsl* **15:**105–108.

50. **Williams PP.** 2010. Culture of blood bank products, Procedure 13.13. *In* Garcia LH (ed), *Clinical Microbiology Procedures Handbook*, 3rd ed. American Society for Microbiology, Washington, DC.

51. **Larone DH.** 2011. *Medically Important Fungi. A Guide to Identification*, 5th ed. American Society for Microbiology, Washington, DC.

52. **Goldmann DA, Pier GB.** 1993. Pathogenesis of infections related to intravascular catheterization. *Clin Microbiol Rev* **6:**176–192.

53. **Liñares J, Sitges-Serra A, Garau J, Pérez JL, Martín R.** 1985. Pathogenesis of catheter sepsis: a prospective study with quantitative and semiquantitative cultures of catheter hub and segments. *J Clin Microbiol* **21:**357–360.

54. **Maki DG.** 1980. Sepsis associated with infusion therapy, p 207–253. *In* Karan S (ed), *Controversies in Surgical Sepsis*. Praeger, New York, NY.

55. **Simor AE, Roberts FJ, Smith JA.** 1988. Cumitech 23, Infections of the Skin and Subcutaneous Tissues. *Coordinating ed*, Smith JA. American Society for Microbiology, Washington, DC.

56. **Swartz MN.** 1990. Cellulitis and superficial infections, p 796–807. *In* Mandell GL (ed), *Principles and Practices of Infectious Diseases*, 3rd ed. Churchill Livingstone, London, United Kingdom.

57. **Gray LD, Fedorko DP.** 1992. Laboratory diagnosis of bacterial meningitis. *Clin Microbiol Rev* **5:**130–145.

58. **Ray CG, Smith JA, Wasilauskas BL, Zabransky R.**1993. Cumitech 14A, Laboratory Diagnosis of Central Nervous System Infections. *Coordinating ed*, Smith JA. American Society for Microbiology, Washington, DC.

59. **Tunkel AR, Scheld WM.** 1993. Pathogenesis and pathophysiology of bacterial meningitis. *Clin Microbiol Rev* **6:**118–136.

60. **Waites KB, Saubolle MA, Talkington DF, Moser SA, Baselski V.** 2006. Cumitech 10A. Laboratory Diagnosis of Upper Respiratory Tract Infections. *Coordinating ed*, Sharp SE. American Society for Microbiology, Washington, DC.

61. **Baker AS, Paton B, Haaf J.** 1989. Ocular infections: clinical and laboratory considerations. *Clin Microbiol Newsl* **11:**97–101.

62. **Gilligan PH, Janda JM, Karmali MA, Miller JM.**1992. Cumitech 12A. Laboratory Diagnosis of Bacterial Diarrhea. *Coordinating ed*, Nolte FS. American Society for Microbiology, Washington, DC.

63. **Bannister ER.** 1993. *Clostridium difficile* and toxin detection. *Clin Microbiol Newsl* **15:**121–123.

64. **Cohen SH, Gerding DN, Johnson S, Kelly CP, Loo VG, McDonald LC, Pepin J, Wilcox MH, Society for Healthcare Epidemiology of America, Infectious Diseases Society of America.** 2010. Clinical practice guidelines for *Clostridium difficile* infection in adults: 2010 update by the society for healthcare epidemiology of America (SHEA) and the infectious diseases society of America (IDSA). *Infect Control Hosp Epidemiol* **31:**431–455.

65. **Harris JC, Dupont HL, Hornick RB.** 1972. Fecal leukocytes in diarrheal illness. *Ann Intern Med* **76:**697–703.

66. **Carr DT, Karlson AG, Stilwell GG.** 1967. A comparison of cultures of induced sputum and gastric washings in the diagnosis of tuberculosis. *Mayo Clin Proc* **42:**23–25.

67. **Van Enk RA, Thompson KD.** 1990. Microbiologic analysis of amniotic fluid. *Clin Microbiol Newsl* **12:**169–172.

68. **Linscott AL.** 2016. Collection, transport, and manipulation of clinical specimens and initial laboratory concerns Procedure 2.1. *In* Leber A (ed), *Clinical Microbiology Procedures Handbook*, 4th ed. American Society for Microbiology, Washington, DC.

69. **Haley LD, Trandel J, Coyle MB.** 1980. Cumitech 11, Practical Methods for Culture and Identification of Fungi in the Clinical Microbiology Laboratory. *Coordinating ed*, Sherris JC. American Society for Microbiology, Washington, DC.

70. **Sharp SE, Robinson A, Saubolle M, Santa Cruz M, Carroll K, Baselski V.** 2004. Cumitech 7B, Laboratory Diagnosis of Lower Respiratory Tract Infections. *Coordinating ed*, Sharp SE. American Society for Microbiology, Washington, DC.

71. **McCarter YS, Burd EM, Hall GS, Zervos M.** 2009. Cumitech 2C. Laboratory Diagnosis of Urinary Tract Infections. *Coordinating ed*, Sharp SE. American Society for Microbiology, Washington, DC.

72. **Versalovic J, Carroll KC, Funke G, Jorgensen JH, Landry ML, Warnock DW (ed).** 2011. *Manual of Clinical Microbiology*, 10th ed. American Society for Microbiology, Washington, DC.

73. **Gleaves CA, Hodinka RL, Johnston SLG, Swierkosz EM.** 1994. Cumitech 15A, Laboratory Diagnosis of Viral Infections. *Coordinating ed*, Baron EJ. American Society for Microbiology, Washington, DC.

74. **Cherry JD, Miller MJ.** 1992. Use of the virology laboratory, p 2363–2369. *In* Feigin RD, Cherry JD (ed), *Textbook of Pediatric Infectious Diseases*, 3rd ed. The W B Saunders Co, Philadelphia, PA.

75. **Chonmaitree T, Baldwin CD, Lucia HL.** 1989. Role of the virology laboratory in diagnosis and management of patients with central nervous system disease. *Clin Microbiol Rev* **2:**1–14.

76. **Christensen ML.** 1989. Human viral gastroenteritis. *Clin Microbiol Rev* **2:**51–89.

77. **Hedberg CW, Osterholm MT.** 1993. Outbreaks of food-borne and waterborne viral gastroenteritis. *Clin Microbiol Rev* **6:**199–210.

78. **Shimizu RY, Grimm F, Garcia LS, Deplazes P.** 2011. Specimen collection, transport, and processing: parasitology, p 2047–2063. *In* Versalovic J, Carroll KC, Funke G, Jorgensen JH, Landry ML, Warnock DW (ed), *Manual of Clinical Microbiology*, 10th ed. American Society for Microbiology, Washington, DC.

79. **Nanduri J, Kazura JW.** 1989. Clinical and laboratory aspects of filariasis. *Clin Microbiol Rev* **2:**39–50.

80. **Clinical and Laboratory Standards Institute.** 2000. *M15-A. Laboratory Diagnosis of Blood-borne Parasitic Diseases; Approved Guideline.* Clinical and Laboratory Standards Institute, Villanova, PA.

81. **Clinical and Laboratory Standards Institute.** 2005. *M28-A2. Procedures for the Recovery and Identification of Parasites From the Intestinal Tract; Approved Guideline; Second informational supplement.* Clinical and Laboratory Standards Institute, Villanova, PA.

# Index